AF387421

PERMISSION *to* HEAL

PERMISSION *to* HEAL

REBUILDING STRENGTH
for WARRIORS, ATHLETES, *and* HIGH PERFORMERS

PRIME HALL
FORMER U.S. MARINE RAIDER

WILEY

Library of Congress Cataloging-in-Publication Data is Available:

ISBN 9781394428618 (Cloth)
ISBN 9781394428625 (ePUB)
ISBN 9781394428632 (ePDF)

Cover Design: Wiley
Cover Image: baona/Getty Images
Author Photo: Warrior Angels Foundation
Printed and bound by CPI Group (UK) Ltd, Croydon, CR0 4YY
C9781394428618_100626

To anyone who was killed in action or ended up taking their own lives as result of their experience in the war on terror.

Life's a dance

you learn as you go

Sometimes you lead

Sometimes you follow

Don't worry about the things that you don't know

Life's a dance

you learn as you go

Writing in loving memory of Dan Brown, Shawn Jensen, John Wayne, Dan Smith, and Giorgio Kirylo.

All glory to God, the source of life for all humanity.

Contents

Foreword

There are few people in this world I trust with my life. Fewer still I've grown alongside in battle, in business, and in the depths of personal transformation. Prime Hall is one of them.

We met in the Marine Special Operations Command (MARSOC) Assessment and Selection in 2010 and went through some of the toughest training in the world together. Before we were ever Marine Raiders, we worked as Instructors of Water Survival on base. We were just two young guys just trying to find our path. From there, we went through the Individual Training Course (ITC), starting with 108 candidates and finishing as 2 of the original 16 graduates. For nearly a decade, he served side-by-side at 1st Marine Raider Battalion, going through deployments, combat, personal losses, and growth.

One moment that sticks with me is the 2 kilometer fin swim we had to complete every morning during ITC. If you didn't make the time, you had to redo it until you did. Finning was my weakness. Running was Prime's. So we trained together, pushed each other, found joy and satisfaction in the suffering, and filled in the gaps where the other came up short. That dynamic—iron sharpening iron—was the foundation of everything that came after.

That mindset carried over into civilian life when we built Deep End Fitness and the Underwater Torpedo League. Prime has always been a force of nature. He is relentless, intense, always dreaming big, and pushing boundaries. I've usually been the one making sure those dreams become reality. That's our dynamic: vision and execution, both rooted in sacrifice and trust in each other and the mission of making our vision accessible to the world.

But what I respect most about Prime isn't just his work ethic or how far he's pushed his mind and body. It's the evolution. From operator to leader, from warrior to husband and father. He's still got that fire, but now it's aimed at building others up—helping people confront fear, find confidence, and transform their lives.

This book isn't fluff. It's not a theory. It's Prime's journey. It's raw, honest, and hard-earned. He's not writing from a mountaintop. He's still in the trenches, doing the work. And that's what makes it real.

Proud to call him my brother. Proud to build with him. And proud of the mission that he and we're on.

Never above you. Never below you. Always beside you.

—Don Tran
Former Marine Raider, cofounder, Deep End Fitness

Introduction

The first friend I had who took his own life was Shawn Jensen. The loss of Shawn has been tremendous and has had a huge impact on my life. Ever since that happened, subconsciously, I have been trying to figure out how he got to that point. Since then, I've had other friends commit suicide, and I personally was at that emotional cliff of taking my own life years later. When you look into the statistics, especially among certain demographics, the numbers are staggering.

When I committed to addressing the impact of my traumas and working toward healing, I was in such a dark, bad place that I could never have known that one day I would be sharing my journey so publicly with other people on long-form podcasts, while speaking to groups about my businesses, and in coaching sessions with professional athletes and high-performing individuals. And now in *Permission to Heal*.

Knowing many strong, vibrant high-performing people who aren't here anymore because they committed suicide has been driving me to find answers and offer my experiences to others, so anyone struggling can find healing and get their life back into a powerful, rewarding flow. Facing this challenge has given me a deeper understanding of how I made my way back to finding inner peace in life, and it is why I feel it is important to share my story.

As I began to break the silence of my experiences and share with my family and those within my communities, the response I have received has been overwhelming. The amount of people who have confided in me about their own experiences or told me how my sharing helped them face their own traumas, depression, or other life hardships such as loss and grief has both humbled me and opened my eyes.

As these conversations kept coming up, it became clear to me that trauma comes in many forms, has many faces, and is often buried very deep. It's experienced by humans young and old. Few, if any, escape this life without some lived experience of it. It also became clear that conventional approaches that are standard and popular in our culture and that did not work for me often don't work for others in ways that lead to lasting change or healing. This tends to leave people frustrated, isolated, hopeless, and in great pain while fighting shame, stigma, or social pressure to conform to cultural norms and expectations.

There is no shame in speaking up and reclaiming your life so you can live fully empowered. Speaking up could be asking for help, which I've realized is one of the hardest things. Speaking up can also be simply putting words to your experiences, verbally expressing something that has been bothering you, or having a conversation with somebody you need to talk to, like reconnecting with an estranged family member, for example.

In writing *Permission to Heal*, my commitment is to share the perspective I've gained through my journey with openness and vulnerability in the effort of helping destigmatize these conversations. I believe we must normalize speaking up and asking for help when needed. If you want a better way forward in your life, you must actively seek it. I'm specifically writing for anyone dealing with depression, anxiety, or trauma and who is seeking healing, which may resonate most with veterans or others operating in or adjusting from rigid institutions. I'm also writing for anyone who wants to move their life forward in a more positive direction. What I have learned is that there is always a way forward—regardless of where you've been, or what you've suffered. I'm here to remind you that you are not alone.

It's important to be equipped if you are committed to facing your past, trauma, depression, anxiety, or any extreme hardship. Or simply looking to grow, improve, and live up to your highest potential. There can be something unsettling about revisiting certain moments in life that shaped you and led you to where you are today and it's important to have patience for yourself, a plan to follow, trusted support, and sometimes professional or medical help, depending on the level of trauma you have encountered.

It can be difficult to know how and where to start. While the methods and paths that I've found to work best for me in pulling me from my darkest times may not be mainstream or comfortable, they are simple, structured, and holistic. They are based in science, lean heavily on nature, biology, and systems. Best approached with an open mind and open heart.

Throughout the book, I include tools, frameworks, and resources that helped me shift my own pain into purpose and losses into wins. And in the back, I link to a full list of exercises, resources, and organizations that I recommend based on proven results and impact I've either experienced myself or witnessed in others. One that is immediately there for you is the National Suicide Prevention Lifeline, which offers services to talk to a skilled counselor.

If you are feeling distressed, need to speak with a counselor, and are considering joining a martial arts community, please call 1-800-273-8255.

CHAPTER 1

Swimming Upstream

I was born in 1984, a year that doesn't feel so distant until you realize how much has changed since then. The world was in motion: technology accelerating, culture shifting, noise everywhere. But I wasn't aware of any of that. What shaped me wasn't the world "out there," it was what was happening behind closed doors at home.

I was born in the Piney Woods of East Texas, which felt like the middle of nowhere. When I was between one and two, my family moved from Piney Woods to Corpus Christi/North Padre Island along the coast of the Gulf of Mexico. We moved there because my dad's parents lived in Corpus Christi. Being near my grandparents ended up being very beneficial for me. The beach and water aren't what usually come to mind when you think of Texas, but North Padre Island is a popular destination along the coast for family vacations, surfing, spring break, and water sports enthusiasts.

Revisiting childhood evokes a lot for a person, and it's been a critical part of my healing and personal growth. On the surface, you might have thought that I had a normal childhood. I played in the soccer league, went to school, and had plenty of friends. Some of these early friends are still in my life today. The reality was that things at home and my relationship with my parents were extremely difficult. Addictions run deep in my family, on both sides. Most days, my mom and dad were trying to get by and deal with their own issues. They argued frequently and eventually divorced. I also have a younger sister, Carly, who was born four years and four days after me.

Siblings often witness the best and the worst, and that was no exception for us.

My dad was often away, but his dog was a constant presence. He raised pit bulls and kept one dog, whom he named Bob Barker, after the host of *The Price Is Right*. Bob Barker was always protective, especially when my mom was out walking. He was an attack dog. One time he got out of our fence and attacked our neighbor's dog and killed it and then attacked the neighbor and bit her. After that he had to be put down.

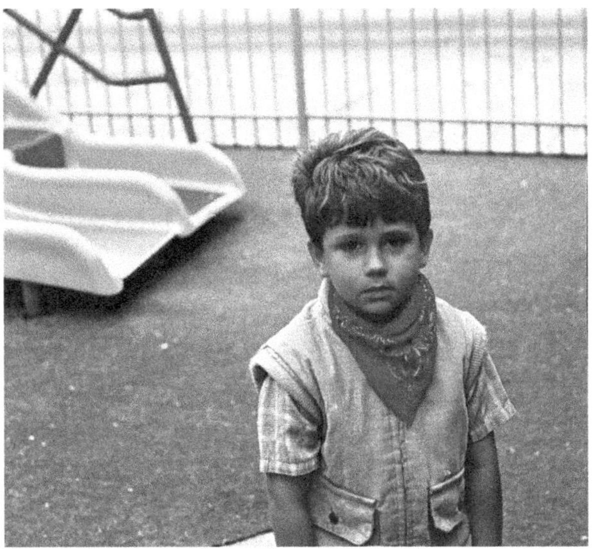

Prime's Younger Years in Corpus Christi

Breakdowns and Breakthroughs

I talk a lot about breakdowns and breakthroughs because time and again, I have seen a breakdown act as a catalyst for a breakthrough. These moments can be critical for healing and finding flow. I've observed this in myself and in many of the highest-performing individuals I've known, served alongside, or coached. I know that if you can just push through the breakdown that growth, breakthroughs and flow often wait on the other side. It requires humility, a willingness to approach the lesson, a commitment to do the work, or sometimes, simply the act of surrender.

One of the sources of abundance from these years was the relationship I built with both sets of grandparents. My maternal grandparents were Nana Joy and Papa, while my father's parents were Grandma Barbara and Grandpa Ralph.

Given the numerous challenges my mom and dad faced in their own lives, my grandparents played a crucial role in helping raise me.

Nana Joy was the disciplinarian and didn't tolerate any disrespect. She had strict standards for behavior when you were in her presence, and she never wavered from those standards. One of the ways Nana Joy showed love was through accountability. Papa was incredibly loving and always there for me when I needed support. He was a successful builder and architect. They set a remarkable example for me and have been pillars of support through some of the toughest times I've faced. I mention them frequently in this book. They laid a foundation for my life that stands to this day.

Grandpa Ralph, my dad's father, was a successful real estate attorney who retired young. He served as the attorney for the Howard Edward Butt, HEB Stores. I inherited one main element of my foundation, my affinity for water and the pool, from Grandma Barbara. She was a wild spirit and a big drinker. She was fond of parties and wasn't afraid to raise her voice. She was also a synchronized swimmer. I grew up going to the pool with her, and from the early days of my childhood, the water has consistently been my sanctuary.

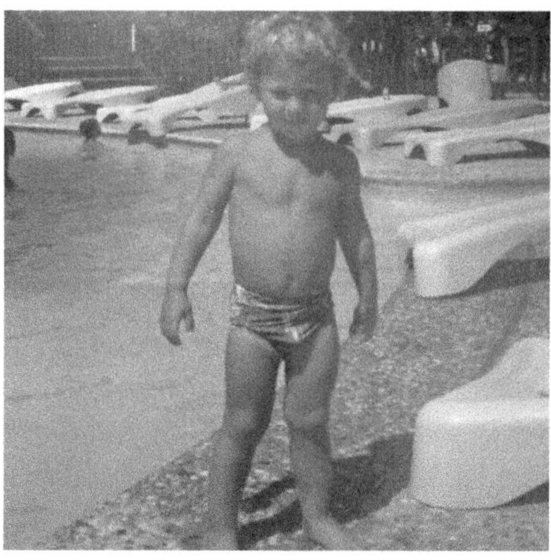

1988 Swimsuit Competitions with My
Grandma Barbara in Corpus Christi, Texas

My memories of being at the pool and engaging in water sports date back to my early years, participating in swimsuit competitions at Grandma Barbara's neighborhood pool. In high school, I served drinks by resort pools to college students flocking to South Padre Island for spring break. Further down the road I underwent training for and served as a Marine Raider. In my professional journey, I cofounded Deep End Fitness and Underwater Torpedo League with Don Tran. Through these experiences I've been able to train countless high-performing individuals and world-class athletes in underwater exercises, preparing them for the most demanding competitions and peak performances of their lives. It's been awe-inspiring to witness the performance transformations that can happen in just a few hours or a day at the pool when one follows a structured process.

Brian Trauma, the First Incident

Brain trauma is a recurring theme in my story. I first experienced it at a young age but only later came to understand its lasting impacts and the side effects on my life.

When I was six and a half, the house we lived in had an iron gate at the front, which was attractive for a kid who wanted to climb up. Once you climbed up on top of the fence, there was a roof on one side and a brick wall in front of it that was about 7 feet tall.

One day while climbing to the top, my mom spotted me and yelled a warning to be careful. Moments later, I lost my grip and fell hard, landing on my head. The impact resulted in a linear fracture across my skull. I blacked out from the fall and was immediately rushed to hospital.

Thankfully, there was no internal bleeding, but the consequences were serious. My skull remained soft, essentially mush for a full year, which meant I was restricted from many of the activities that I loved, such as not playing with friends at recess or participating in physical education classes. It took a full year for my skull to harden again, gradually regaining its solidity.

That year and its limitations left a mark far deeper than the fracture. I remember the isolation, the feeling of being different, like an outcast and left out. Back then, there was less understanding and accommodation for individual needs. There was less sensitivity to nuanced needs and a lot of generalization. So, during recess, I would find myself isolated on the sidelines or grouped with the teacher and the children deemed "special needs," separated from the "regular" and seemingly higher-functioning kids.

This was my introduction to traumatic brain injury. Beyond the physical pain of severe headaches, the social repercussions affected me, too.

Looking back on that period, I recognize a significant breakthrough. From this young age, I began honing my skills in observing group dynamics from a vantage point of detachment, enhancing my emotional intelligence. Additionally, it offered me early training in challenging and navigating beyond societal norms and expectations, what I reference as *the Matrix*. This isolation enabled me to start to break away from the pack and groupthink.

The Concept of Flow

My initial understanding of flow came from my intensive involvement in swimming. The two core biomechanics of swimming are minimizing friction and maximizing propulsion. I've dedicated countless hours to underwater performance training, refining athletes' forms to eliminate drag and enhance flow through their arm and leg actions, body positioning, and glide efficiency. When you are underwater, especially while holding your breath, energy conservation is paramount, promoting streamlined, efficient movements. Reducing drag and adding flow is the essence of "economy of motion."

Through training over 15,000 athletes, including military personnel, our team at Deep End Fitness gained a deeper understanding of flow and drag. Collaborating with world champions and elite athletes across various sports, I helped them identify and remove obstacles limiting their performance, resulting in them unlocking a new flow state.

Expanding the Concept of Flow Beyond the Pool

In training people in the pool, this question keeps coming up over and over again: How can we apply these principles to enhance flow and reduce drag in all aspects of life? How can we increase flow in our personal lives? Water serves as a microcosm of life, reflecting how we respond to stress and challenges. By focusing on unlocking flow, I've witnessed numerous breakthroughs in relationships, mindset shifts (from fixed to open), and increased positive coping mechanisms.

Our methodology at Deep End Fitness (DEF), F.R.E.E., centers on unlocking flow:

- **Focus:** Maintaining concentration and present-moment awareness
- **Relaxation:** Reducing tension and anxiety, promoting ease of movement
- **Economy of motion:** Optimizing movement efficiency and energy conservation
- **Efficient breathing:** Ensuring adequate oxygen intake and controlled breathing patterns

The F.R.E.E. operating system is a complete tool to support self-regulation and recovery. These techniques are crucial for underwater training and can be applied to various life domains. When we prioritize our recovery, we have the ability to better regulate ourselves and our performance can be more sustainable.

Additional Mechanisms of Flow

Flow is not limited to physical performance. It can encompass self-realization, self-actualization, breakthroughs, love, joy, and fulfilling relationships. Reducing friction or drag, both mental and physical, is essential for unlocking flow. In the military, instructors often use the phrase "high speed, low drag" to emphasize the importance of streamlined action and minimal resistance. Releasing emotional drag can also play a significant role in enhancing flow.

Integrating Flow into Daily Life

By incorporating these principles into our daily lives, we can optimize our performance, enhance our well-being, and cultivate a greater sense of ease and fulfillment. Whether in our work, relationships, or personal pursuits, the pursuit of flow can lead to greater success, happiness, and overall life satisfaction.

I have found that to effectively invite flow into daily life, it's important to look back to childhood and the early moments we experienced that shaped our lives and view of the world. Sometimes things from early in life can cause drag. We may not be aware of these things. Other times we may be hyperaware of them. We are given the gift of innocence as a child. Family discord, situational trauma, and world events can interrupt our healthy emotional development, which can follow us throughout our lives until we're able to realize and deal with it. I avoided doing this until later in life, when everything felt like it was crumbling around me and I had no other choice.

CHAPTER 2

Reframing Pain into Purpose

Predators and Pain

When I was eight, we moved to a different part of Corpus Christi, on the south side of town. Just outside my bedroom on the side of the house was a bunch of plants and shrubs landscaped around the window. Unexpectedly, this landscape became the perfect hiding place for a predator lurking in the shrubs and plants. To be honest, I blocked out and suppressed most memories of this traumatic time. They became a buried pain deep within my mind and soul. It wasn't until undergoing intense therapy following wartime experiences that these memories resurfaced, enabling me to confront and process them.

The timeline is blurred in my memory. I don't remember how long after we moved into this new house this all started, but a voyeuristic "peeping Tom" frequently hid in the bushes outside my window, secretly watching me in my room. Sometimes his presence felt surreal, like the boogie man, but soon enough he would become very real—with distinct sounds of tapping and breathing on my window. When I spotted him for the first time, I remember going to get my parents. My dad pulled out his gun and went outside to confront the intruder, but the guy had vanished. This scenario repeated itself many, many times. For years, I would sleep in my closet. I wouldn't even be in the vicinity of my bed, hoping the man wouldn't see me. Whenever it got overwhelming, I would knock on the wall and if my dad was there, he would come to my room or go outside, but he never caught him. My family didn't believe me for years, stripping me of any sense of real emotional or psychological validation.

Around this time, caller ID became available, and we had one plugged in beside our landline phone. I started receiving phone calls from an unidentified number. Picking up, I would only hear a man's heavy breathing on the other end of the line. It scared me every time. Despite my efforts to compartmentalize, various bizarre experiences continued to happen. Occasionally, while I was riding my bike during the day, I was followed by a car. Fight or flight kicked in, and I rode my bike as fast as I could to get somewhere in hiding where passing cars couldn't see me. One of the places where I felt safe was the park all the way down at the end of my street. This park had its own share of troubles, but I felt safer there somehow. The reality was, I didn't feel truly safe anywhere, except when I was with my grandparents. As a result of coping with the situation without any communication or support, I developed a heightened sense of awareness, as I tried to deal with the situation while operating in survival mode.

This went on for four to five years. Until one night, while I was asleep in the closet, my parents finally caught the predator at my window. My dad ran out and chased him all the way to the park. Once my parents caught him, they cut down the trees he would hide in, installed security lights and it stopped being a problem. But then a few months later my parents divorced, and it was quickly forgotten as our family went in different directions. I didn't realize how much this lack of validation and protection bothered me until years later. Through part of my healing process, I took on a victim mentality and dealt with a lot of anger about why I endured such suffering and fear as an innocent child. This has become especially pronounced as I raise my own children, because of the immense love I have for them, and the responsibility I feel to protect them and my wife and loved ones across my family tree.

When my parents' divorce finally happened, it was a relief for us. However, it seemed to affect my sister much more than it did me. Our relationship faced some serious rough patches as we both struggled to cope and adapt. My relationship with each of my parents was rocky at different times. I have made significant efforts with forgiveness and personal growth to be on positive terms with both of my parents today. As a family, we've worked to break patterns and habits that have hindered us for generations. Some of my most challenging breakdowns were triggered by how my family functioned. But so were some of my most profound breakthroughs.

The pain I experienced at home was paving the way for my resilience and future purpose.

Action Figures and Purpose

When the peeping Tom first started, my first instinct was to tell my parents. But when that didn't make the man or the problem go away, I adapted the best I could to handle what I was experiencing. As humans, this is what we do. It's not always easy to figure out the root of why and when we start adapting in little ways that grow bigger and more problematic later. But often, our coping mechanisms can be traced back to early childhood.

As kids, we're not equipped yet to solve these kinds of problems. And when our environments don't help us work through the problems, or worse, the situations are unsafe, we will do whatever is necessary to adapt and survive. Especially at a young age.

My best breakthrough from this time of pain was developing high adaptability in response to my circumstances and for the challenges I would face later in what I think of as "life school." I also look back at this period as early preparation for my future in military school, which laid the foundation for my future training for and time as a Marine Raider.

One way I adapted for these years was to always sleep in the closet. I did this to remain outside of the viewpoint of the window—especially at night. There were lights in the closet, but I always wanted to have them off so the man couldn't see me. I tried to make it as comfortable as possible so I felt safe enough to sleep. I considered it a huge win that I never had to make my bed, ever, because I never slept in it. When I had friends over to spend the night, it became a game we played to hide from the windows. It almost felt like we were playing a military game, trying not to be seen and avoiding an enemy. It felt like hanging out behind enemy lines.

On TV at the time, they targeted marketing to young boys with action figures in all these fighting stances. Collecting these was my hobby. I had eight shelves on each side of my bedroom full of them. On each shelf, I had different action figures set up and on display. My room was always set up perfectly. But I never really touched them or played with them. I treated it more like a museum. The shelves were in direct view of the window, helping block the view to my closet and giving me a sense of protection.

I did not think consciously about these details at the time or in the following years. I didn't want to remember them and kept them suppressed for many years. I don't know that I would have ever been able to pull these memories out if I didn't have professional help years later when I was in a treatment called Rapid Response Therapy for trauma from war. This treatment was enlightening, helping me go from being very turned off from my emotions, like a total robot, to reclaiming my sensitivity to the world around me and the people in my life. Even my sensitivity to strangers was incredibly high. I share more about this later.

Through conversations, experience, and learning, I realize increasingly that so many people have emotional and sexual trauma they have never dealt with. When somebody said to me, "Prime, you had a sexual predator," it hit me differently. At first, I denied it. I would respond, "No, I wasn't touched or assaulted physically." But they said, "Yes, that's exactly what it was." We downplay our experiences all the time. We often compare it to somebody else who we think had it worse than us. Like my problems weren't as bad as this person or that person, and we try to undermine or discredit our own experiences. And while there are varying degrees of trauma, it's not honoring yourself to use this as an excuse to not address what needs to be addressed.

If we have these things eating away at us, we aren't able to have our oxygen mask on in life and be the best version of ourselves. At some point, we must face, address, and integrate them. If we don't, it's proven that these issues come back and rear up in ugly ways, often repeating the cycle of abuse. This is especially true with people who had physical or sexual assault growing up and buried it. Or often, somebody has a family member who had something traumatic happen to them. Then they went on to repeat it by doing the same thing to somebody else, keeping the cycle going.

Acknowledging, addressing, and integrating the experiences and healing are very important. My advice is that as you begin to do the work and approach versus avoid your past be aware that it can bring up powerful, even volatile emotions. After the specific treatment that resurfaced it all to my mind, my sensitivity to everything was extremely high.

So, it's important that you have the right people around you during this time. Like an Ultimate Fighting Championship fighter has their corners offering support, strategy, and encouragement, and coaches in their corner for a fight, you need to do this in life if you want to unlock your highest potential. It's equally important to cut any toxic ties, relationships, and habits as much as possible. And let go of things that keep you stuck in old patterns or in negative mind-sets. It's so important to have a safe space with trusted support around you as you do the work to face it all. Be it family or professionals. When you have the right people around you, it's scientifically proven to lower the stress response.

Facing things and dealing with obstacles can be extremely stressful, but sometimes, the only way to the other side is straight through the obstacle. One time, I was with Steve Magness, who has done a lot of research on resilience, at a human performance conference in Texas. I like and recommend his book, *Do Hard Things: Why We Get Resilience Wrong and the Surprising Science of Real Toughness*. In it, he tells a story about fear inoculation, in which scientists conducted a stress response study and monitored the fear response of participants. Participants were exposed to something they were afraid of, without any support system around them. Then they did the same stressful thing, but the participants had their support system present this time. The difference in stress response was significant when the support system was present. When you have a support system you can move through and deal with much more than you could on your own.

Certain ways of looking at this process can help keep you on track. Specifically, challenge yourself as quickly as possible to look at the obstacles in front of you as opportunities in order to reframe them into something positive that will work for you as you move forward. It is also important to create a process to self-regulate and deal with the things that come up, so that you can be prepared with practices to help integrate.

In my life, I've reframed my story from "having a predator as a child was the worst thing that ever happened" to "dealing with a predator as a young child was the training that set me up for success for my entire life." It wasn't clear that my traumas came from so far back in my life. Brain trauma and post-traumatic stress—sure, that makes sense. But sometimes, it's not clear, and there are signs that point to something deeper.

Signs and symptoms of trauma or unresolved problems are different for every person. They may look different for you than for me. For me, there were some red flags that are very clear now:

- All relationships struggling and difficult
- Feeling disconnected from any sense of baseline
- Excessively drinking
- Relying on prescription medications
- Living with anxiety and/or depression
- Having invasive and recurring suicidal thoughts

Now more than ever, depression and anxiety have increased across the globe. I currently view depression as a signal that something is seriously out of alignment. When you become aware of whatever is bothering you and you pull it out from being buried, it can be a very uncomfortable process. Having a support system around you as you go through the process is critical. I can't stress this enough.

Suppose you feel like you are getting stuck or going backward, which is not uncommon when you begin to do this work. Look into mechanisms that keep you going and moving forward. Pattern disruption techniques are tools to break up whatever pattern you find yourself stuck in. You can also adopt an approach versus avoid mindset. Once you identify where you are stuck or set back, approach it so you can lean in, process, and move through it. Find healthy and therapeutic coping methods that work for you because coping on some level is part of the process. Last, plan for integration.

I talk more about these mechanisms in greater depth throughout the book and in the resources section so that you can have an arsenal of tools to apply for yourself or investigate more.

CHAPTER 3

Safe Spaces and Mentors

Isolation and Finding Safe Spaces

When you have issues at home, problems are likely to show up in other areas of life, too. As a kid, that's usually school. In the fourth and fifth grades I began to find my own solutions for the stuff I was dealing with, such as if I was having problems with the teachers. I learned recently that my mom went to parent-teacher meetings in my fourth- and fifth-grade years, and both years, she found I had different teachers than when I started. My initial teacher was awful both years, and I advocated for myself and got switched to the nicer teacher both years in a row. Post-military I had to fight my way through a victim mindset again and get curious about how this period shaped me and how I coped so that I could begin to work through and integrate these experiences. I realize now that was me starting to claim my agency and independence.

One primary way I coped in this stage of life was by finding or creating safe environments for myself. Safe physical, emotional, and psychological spaces are a big deal to me. Aside from seeking safe spaces as a child, finding them as an adult in war was a matter of life and death. I found ways to find or create them when I was young, and I continue to prioritize them today. Creating a safe space is critical to drive performance, communication, and resilience.

Growing up in Corpus Christi, my bike became an essential avenue for finding safe spaces. It wasn't uncommon for me to run away from home and ride my bike all the way across town to my grandparents' house. I would stay with them as often as I could. I always had those little BMX-style bikes, and I got into riding them with one of my best friends, John, and his younger brother, Price. I stayed with John and Price often as well. Their parents were divorced, and they lived with their mom. She was a lawyer and worked a lot, which left us to do our own thing. We rode our bikes everywhere.

There are also many times when I recall seeking and finding safety or protection in unusual places, such as the times that I would ride my bike to the park at the end of our street to avoid the man from the window when I thought he was following me around in his car. This park had a lot of trouble going on, a lot of gang activity happening. I never saw anyone get shot or anything like that, but there was a lot of fighting, people getting jumped, and other crazy, violent things. Being near it was both a good thing and a bad thing for me. To be allowed to be part of the park, I had to get jumped first, an initiation of sorts. I saw this as a good thing because I could go to the park, and I didn't think the man would be there. I thought he would be eaten alive at that park if he dared to show up. I was safe but not safe. I didn't know it yet, but this was also preparation for military school and later, the military itself.

Living Alone and Scarcity

About the time I was heading into high school, I moved in with my dad. But the reality was that he was never there because he was living with his girlfriend. He would occasionally check on me, but day after day, I was completely alone and on my own at home. I didn't have rules to follow or adults watching after me. I was just a young teenager, and after the issues with my peeping Tom, I still sometimes got freaked out and had to figure out ways to fight through those moments. I kept it all to myself and never talked about it with my grandparents or friends at school.

I lived in pure survival mode in my freshman and sophomore years of high school. High school was a lot to deal with, especially without any guidance. And it was hard to go home to an empty house after school at night. I didn't have anyone to talk to about what I was facing at school. I was figuring things out the hard way, hitting my head against the wall over and over again. I would go to school, speak out against the older kids, and sometimes get beat up for it.

I have an August birthday, so I was always a year or two younger than everyone else in my class. So, when I started high school at 13, turning 14 years old, I was not very big in comparison to my peers and ended up being hazed by some of the seniors. Freshman initiation is a thing that goes on at certain schools, and I didn't understand why this behavior was acceptable to anyone. But by this point, I knew how to stand up for myself after being in the park so much, so when the seniors gave me trouble, I would resist and fight back— and they did not like this. I wasn't having or taking any of it and resisted completely. This resistance created a lot of conflict, and this conflict would not let up. All year long, I got into fights and had problems with the same seniors. After every incident, I found myself looking back and saying what the fuck was this for? What am I doing here trying to prove myself to these spoiled kids just looking for an ego trip, living for some popularity contest?

Since I didn't know how to cope or get external help, I created systems in my mind to get through those moments. I convinced myself that I could not be hurt—that if I got hit or jumped, it would not phase me. I told myself that these guys could do whatever they wanted to do; it was impossible to hurt me. I'm not going to feel it. I will turn it off. I may not have been as physically mature as everyone else was yet, but mentally, I had been through a lot and had found ways to adapt and cope. I was in a constant state of fight or flight, and I was quick to fight for myself.

The Power of Mentors

My grandparents, Bill and Joy (Nana and Papa), really stepped up about this time and ultimately helped change the course of my life. They wanted me to have experiences and opened the world to me. They would often take me on trips, which I looked forward to every time. We went to places like Mexico, Las Vegas, and New York. These are some of my better memories, and they taught me a lot and exposed me to new things. Their involvement showed me the power of mentors, and I leaned on their support many times. I encourage everyone to identify positive mentors and find ways to mentor others.

One time, my grandparents planned a summer trip to San Antonio. When they picked me up for the trip, they realized I was living alone. When they discovered this, they were shocked and became increasingly concerned. They found the conditions unacceptable.

One day on this vacation, we were at the mall, and I saw some other kids there in what looked like military uniforms. It turns out the Texas Military Institute for teenagers is in San Antonio. I mentioned how cool it would be to do something like that, and my grandparents took note of my interest. When they took me home after this trip and looked more fully into the reality of my living situation, they started asking more questions. Then they found a solution—fast. They asked if I would like to go on a tour of the Marine Military Academy (MMA), located next to South Padre Island. I loved everything that I saw there. It was such an amazing campus. An expensive, high-level boarding school, and my grandparents helped me get enrolled, which led to my first great transformation in life.

The Importance of Integration

I did not always see these moments as transformations. Still, over time, I've learned to reframe and integrate my experiences and lessons from these years.

I could ruminate that I had a stressful and horrible childhood without much support and love and that my innocence was gone at an early age. I could view myself as a victim and complain that nobody else I knew in my neighborhood had the kind of stuff going that I did. I know now that these things are really what put me on a trajectory to military school and ultimately to where I am today.

Understanding your trauma and how it shaped your life and integrating your experiences are two different actions.

Integration takes a lot of intentionality. A coach or mentor can be very helpful when doing this. You do have to integrate once you identify a traumatic event or pain point that you are processing if you truly want to heal. And once you take the initial steps to approach and process that event, it can bring up a lot or even put you back into survival mode.

We've all done things to integrate our experience while operating out of survival mode. However, what we want to do is integrate through a process. You can refine your process along the way. But it's essential to have some kind of process and a plan in place. I go deeper into the topic of integration later in the book, but it's important to get familiar and comfortable with the idea of integration for healing and growth.

Here are some simple questions you can ask yourself as you explore the concept of integration:

- What kind of conversations will create opportunities for you to move through this obstacle?
- Which people in your life are in your corner? Whom can you partner with to lean into and process something that you need to approach?
- Where and with whom do or will you need to set boundaries?
- What's missing right now that would foster integration? (example, accountability, trust, communication, _______)

For many, the pivotal moments of lasting trauma do come from childhood. One powerful integration exercise I was guided through that was very therapeutic and helped a lot was completing a childhood rescue mission. I was instructed to "be" myself now as an adult, and observe myself as a child, in the vulnerable or traumatic moments from childhood, and then enact a rescue of that child version of myself.

So 30 years later, I was able to visualize and deeply experience myself as an adult setting my child self free, using a crowbar to rip out a window and conduct a rescue of the younger version of myself who was scared and hiding in my closet. That was a therapeutic and powerful release for me.

What does your childhood rescue mission look like? Even if you had a "good" childhood, that doesn't mean that you don't still have a childhood rescue mission. What was missing? Was it too easy or was it too hard? How does the childhood version of yourself need to be rescued, protected, or spoken to to heal parts of yourself that are still stuck there.

I don't want to pretend or mislead that this is an easy thing to do or a quick process that one exercise can accomplish. I compartmentalized my experiences for so long and didn't begin to process most of these things until much later, after years in the military. Beginning to integrate these experiences from childhood took time and it was difficult. It took many years and many approaches. The last thing I want to do is make anyone think that there is some magical solution. Integration is key and takes time, effort, and patience.

CHAPTER 4

Embracing Transformation

One of the things about looking back in time is how much more clearly you can identify your transformations. Key decisions, choices, and actions that were pivotal in how you grew, changed, and evolved become apparent consciously for the first time.

Day-to-day, certain moments themselves may not seem like such a big deal, but when you reflect over a longer period of time, you can see certain moments that stand out as transformational or recognize patterns that you can learn from. We can also harness awareness of patterns to make healthier transformations and day-to-day choices.

Transformation

One of my Aussie friends, Cinzia, is a meditation guide. One day she explained the process that lobsters go through when they grow. A lobster's shell does not grow. So as the lobster is ready to grow, it gets very uncomfortable in it's now too small shell and must grow a new and bigger shell. They go off alone, under a rock or in a cave, where they can shed the old shell and grow a new shell, before returning into their lobster community. We can look at the transformation that the lobster goes through like a self-transformation process we can go through as humans. Even lobsters go DEEP to find a transformative breakout to create their next life phase!

Are you willing to go into this process and create the shell you need? Or are you constantly staying in your shell that has no more room for growth? Your shell can be the contents of your life, such as the following:

- Beliefs/self-talk
- Who you are around
- Where you live
- What car you drive (material shell)
- What your profession is
- Who your friends are
- Accomplishments or status
- Habits
- Hobbies

These things are your shell. It's not to say all these things are bad or need to go. Taking inventory of which elements of your shell are healthy or not healthy is important for your own self-awareness and for your overall well-being. We should outgrow our shells in certain areas and times in life. When we do, we're going to have to go through transformational processes to build that next shell.

Once the lobster goes through its self-transformation and reenters its lobster community, it looks different and may not fit in how it used to. If you've been finding ways to numb pain or fear or just stay comfortable, your shell may be things that aren't serving you, like alcohol, clubbing, unhealthy habits, relationships, or certain friendships.

It's important to manage your expectations through this process when it comes to others you are surrounded by. When you go through a period of growth and come out on the next level, with a revamped version of your shell, there may be judgment from the people who expect you to look and act the same as you used to. Not everyone has regrown their shell and come out transformed. Sometimes they are still attached to the old shell, still doing the same things you have now outgrown. And you won't fit in anymore. They may judge you as you behave differently, and you might feel misunderstood. But know that growth brings change. Sometimes there are necessary endings and necessary beginnings that come with growth. As one door closes, another one opens.

But as humans, transformations and growth don't have to happen alone or without support. You can also grow in community with others and lean on relationships. The challenge here is to look at your shell and make an assessment on what and how you need to grow. What is the goal that you have, where are you now, and what is the gap you need to fill to reach your goal?

For me, embracing and expressing my emotions and experiencing the emotions of others can be uncomfortable. That's a gap I have wanted to close, so I've been going through some transformational emotional intelligence (EQ) courses. Emotions are not easy to face, and as an extreme introvert, being in groups like that is a constant challenge. I've been working on it for years now and nothing about it feels cool or fun. For somebody who can't swim emotionally it feels like jumping into the deep end of the pool. Going into that room for a three-day course with 100 other people is uncomfortable. It's training and it is built to be a breakthrough opportunity. And my nature is to be resistant. But I've learned that the transformation in my life is worth it. I keep up this effort, whether I'm in resistance or engaged, because I am achieving emotional transformation. I also do things that are physically or mentally challenging to grow in these ways. I do things like jiu jitsu, underwater training, and boxing. It's the same thing, but I'm working on a different part of the shell.

Many people whom I have worked with or coached follow a practice similar to the lobsters; it has been a life-changing experience working with Olympians and world champions. Transformations that take work and effort are the last thing high-level athletes want to do at the end of the day. But these people are actively rebuilding their shells. Those who put in the work are evolving spiritually, mentally, physically, emotionally, and psychologically to unlock their highest levels of potential in all these areas.

If you do the work you will likely experience growth and change in all different ways. As a result, your shell is going to look different from before you leveled up. Before you may have had a soft shell. And now, you have almost a turtle shell. So now, it's going to stand out and look different. You are transforming yourself and figuring out how to turn into the best version of yourself as a person, spouse, athlete, artist, professional, performer, martial artist, or anything else. How are you going to continue to evolve and transform?

You may not know how your evolution will develop or show up, but it's the act of staying in the transformation process that is where the magic happens.

Accountability

On the transformation journey, you must have accountability built in. People fear growth and change. With real transformation, you will feel challenged and vulnerable. Change in our mind feels like danger. It's like messing with our survival. But it's a change in a positive direction, depending on the goal, process, and dedication. Dedication and accountability are the key to positive change and growth.

For instance, my nutrition and fitness coach Mike Lemaire takes accountability very seriously. When we started, he said, "So, on Monday I want to see a photo of you on the scale, and a photo of you with your shirt off."

He did that at the start of the program. Now, the transformation process is really locked in. Then ongoing, every Monday I sent him a photo of me with my shirt off and another of the numbers on the scale reading. He started this for accountability. If there's no accountability worked in, there's not that same amount of commitment. This is a huge principle that applies to many areas.

With boxing and kickboxing. I have videos of myself when I suck, and I put it out there, and I get feedback and it makes me better. That becomes an accountability system.

You can build accountability systems with different things. Beyond fitness, my accountability system is built into every area of my life. For instance, I can bring an idea or scenario in front of my wife, Brittany, so she can analyze it and give me feedback. I use that as an accountability system to unlock performance.

You can go to the gym, and you can go to the pool (or fill in the blank). You can put out, say, 10% effort, and you can get 1% of change. Or you can go, and you can put yourself into training and environments where there is going to be exponential growth, such as with coaches, training partners, healing circles, anything outside of yourself. Because when you have accountability outside of yourself, you will always go further and do more than you can on your own.

For the most challenging goals, I believe there must be accountability outside of yourself to meet your goals and full potential.

For example, if you are running sprints, and you must do this every week, do you think you will have the same effort when you are alone or when you have a team around you or people you are racing against? There's a different level of effort. So how can we incorporate outside accountability more into our life?

The biggest point here is to have an accountability partner—somebody who looks at you and your life and spends time and energy helping you keep track of your goals. That's love and support being shown. Sometimes people get defensive during this process. But ask yourself, Do I need to be defensive or is this person really trying to support me?

Never stop building your new shell. Never stop growing. Build the journey, not the destination. Remember the journey that the lobster goes through transforming and reintegrating with the new shell in the old tribe or finding a new tribe.

Marine Military Academy

I was 15 turning 16 when I got to the Marine Military Academy. I was relieved and happy to be there. The other students were anywhere from the 8th grade to post-high school, so 12 or 13 years old up to about 20 years old. It was not uncommon for people who were having a hard time graduating high school to be sent here by their families to finish. Most people who go to that school are there against their will because they got in trouble, and it was almost like a prison environment.

Going there meant being locked down with a bunch of troublemakers and dangerous kids and young adults. Fights happened all day, every day because we knew we wouldn't get kicked out for fighting. However, at the same time, it was very structured with rules that were enforced and came with a lot of security. This is the main reason why I wanted to go there. It was different for me than other people in that way, because there was no chance of the man from the window watching or following me. I wasn't coming home every day to an empty house with no support, rules, or wondering where my next meal was coming from. Even though there was a lot of intense stuff going on there I felt safer and had a sense of tremendous relief. Somehow I started to live more freely.

The first 30 days were our boot camp. During boot camp, you live in barracks, just like when you join the military. You have a roommate and you share the bathroom with them and two others. Everything is connected in these two-story buildings.

Being there was super action packed. The school is essentially run by the students. There are drill instructors who manage everything, but the cadets really run the system. The students who have been there over time and have shown most leadership are the ones in charge. In an academy like this, however, hazing tends to happen, too. And if you get into a situation like that, you want to establish dominance, because people are going to relentlessly test you in that environment. The last thing you want to show is that you can be run over; otherwise, everyone will try to do that. Like most people there, I got into fights in the first weeks and months inside and outside the barracks. Really it was standing up for yourself and joining in for others whom you want to stand up for.

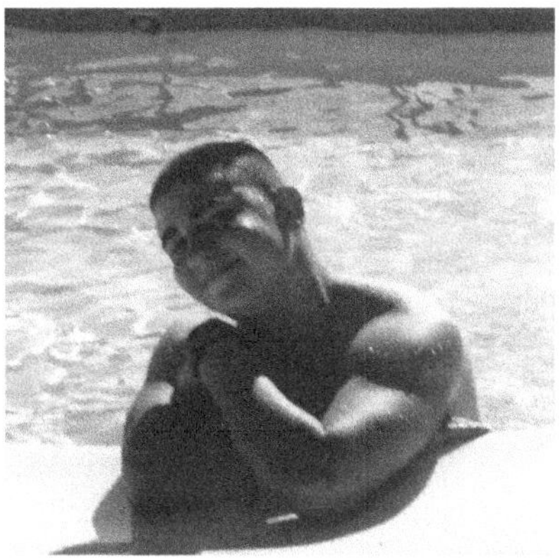

South Padre Island, Texas, During
a Weekend Off from Military
School (2001)

It was a fully secured facility, but my life wasn't all inside of this campus. I constantly hung out at the beach or pools at South Padre Island. In some ways I got the best of both worlds while I was there. I lived at military school, but I had family locally, which meant I could keep my car and spend time with them on the weekends. And sometimes during the week I would find ways to sneak out in the middle of the night with my friends and drive down to Mexico where my roommate's family was from. His family was well off. We would go to stay with his family. They would have these big, crazy events with security guards wearing bulletproof vests. I was a little crazy at this age, so going into these new types of environments was appealing to me and opened my eyes to the world. The richest people in the area, "high society," would be there as well as local newspapers reporting on the parties. The experiences were so different.

A lot of these guys who went on these trips were from politically prominent families. The partying was like nothing I have ever experienced. Even living near Los Angeles later, nothing scratched the surface of the partying that happened in Mexico. Since we were so close to the border, we used to sneak out, party all night, and come back in the morning.

One night we were coming back across the border from Mexico, and one of our friends passed out and was unresponsive. We ended up getting detained. One of the first times I observed the influence of political power was when we were released quickly because one of the guy's dads was politically connected. But we still got caught and got in trouble at school.

I established some cool friends during this time, some of whom I am still close with to this day, like my friend Farid Trad, from Monterrey, Mexico. He lives in Mexico and has a house in San Diego, so I still see him a couple times a year. I've gotten a chance to go back and speak at the military academy a few times to talk to the kids there. I tell the stories of what we did and show pictures of Farid and me, so they know I can relate to what they are going through, and they see somebody out on the other side.

If you had good behavior, they would let you out on Saturday and Sundays for a window of time so you can go out with your friends. But the rule was you had to be in your uniform. And that creates an interesting dynamic, because now you are a target for people who see uniforms and like to call you names or stir up trouble. Sometimes we would get into scuffles when we were off base.

One time I was with my roommate and another friend who had grown up around a Mexican cartel and was a very seasoned person for being just a high school senior. We were walking down the street in our uniforms when some guys drove by and yelled at us disrespectfully.

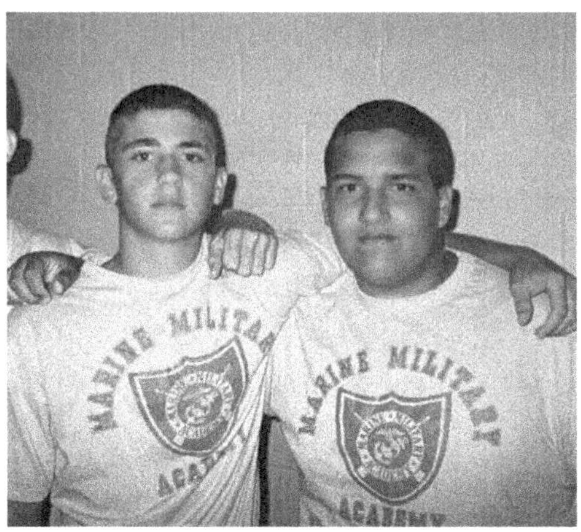

Prime with Farid Trad at Marine Military
Academy in Harlingen, Texas (2001)

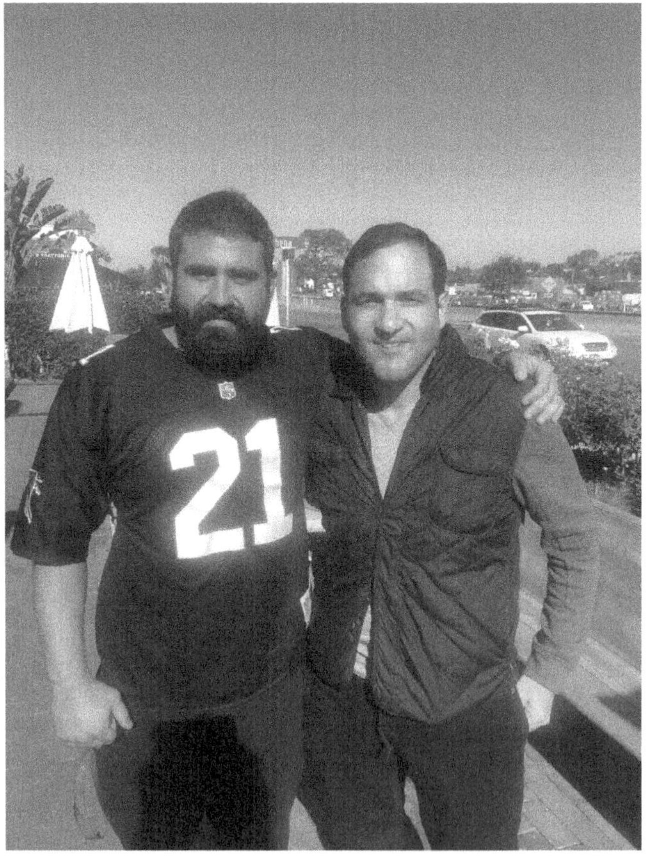

Prime with Farid Trad in San Diego (2022)

When they stopped at a red light just down the road, my friend grabbed one of the riders out of the car and beat him up. At that time, it felt like a moment of street justice, a merit-based thing, where we needed to show that you can't just drive by and call people names unless you are ready to deal with the repercussions of that.

During this time, I got a taste of what life in the military would be like. I learned to lean on my team and friends around me. In some ways, the Marine Military Academy was even more raw than being in the Marine Corps, not from combat, but in the training we had and learning that people depend on you. Later, when in the military itself, it seemed more pro wrestling style. Everything was very loud and there was a lot of screaming in your face. It looks and feels like extreme theatrics. It's meant to prepare and condition you to deal with stress. Military stress tests create adaptations to deal with high-stress, real-world environments.

Humans can adapt to anything with training and preparation. We can go from a first-world country to a war time environment in weeks or a month and adapt to it.

Over time you can have three or five drill instructors in your face, and you can be calm as a cucumber, almost in a meditative state, which prepares for the most extreme real situations so you can be calm and react with a process.

These processes can and should be simple and easy to remember. Such as being able to calm your mind enough in the chaos to perform an OODA loop, a framework used by fighter pilots: observe, orient, decide, act. Fighter pilots can adapt from never flying to be able to process and engage/deconflict with enemy fighter pilots.

Jiu jitsu is another good example. If somebody is on top, in mount, and threatening a choke, but also threatening an arm lock, you must focus on the thing that is most threatening at the time and OODA loop. I provide an OODA loop exercise in the Resources section.

At the end of my first two months at the Marine Military Academy, we had a challenge. The morning that we completed the crucible, or the final event of boot camp, when we had to stay up for an entire night and go through a bunch of challenges, they allowed parents to come. My mom came and I remember her being in awe of how in shape I was, and how much I had learned the military procedures and everything that was part of military school.

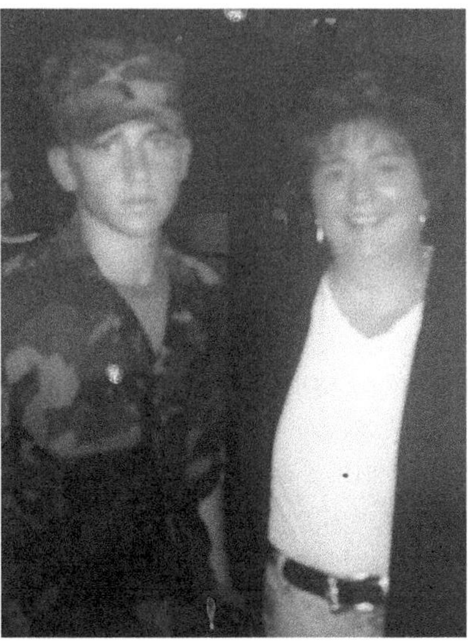

Prime with His Mom After
Finishing Boot Camp at Marine
Military Academy (2001)

Break on Through to the Other Side

After my junior year at the military academy, a lot of my friends were leaving and not coming back. Two of my closer friends from military school passed away. One died in the school year in a skiing incident, and one was shot and killed that summer. I decided I didn't want to go back after that. I also knew it was a very expensive and my grandparents were paying the tuition, so I decided to return to public high school in Corpus Christi for my senior year.

At this point I was about to turn 17, and I was ready for a taste of independence again. My grandparents were on a long vacation in Spain and they let me live at their house. My child support money was coming straight to me via my grandparents as I had a minimal relationship with my dad at that time. I had an allowance, my own car, and a place to stay. This is how my senior year started. Here I was again with no rules, but this time it felt exciting instead of scary. I had a new shell.

My experience in high school was very different this time. Everything about me had transformed and all the things that were hard for me before were easy now. My schoolwork was super easy to complete coming from a military prep school. I was usually able to finish my work in class and never had homework hanging over me. I worked out, doing a lot of strength and conditioning, and learned grappling and fighting training. Plus, I had been in a decent number of fights at military school and knew how to respond if anyone tried to give me trouble.

I gained a lot of confidence and socially things were better, too. Word had gotten around that I had been at military school, and this put a target on me, but in a good way this time. People were more interested in me, how I lived by myself and was independent, able to do whatever I wanted and go where I wanted. And at the same time, I didn't like all the new attention, so I kept to myself and a small circle of friends.

It's not to say that I didn't still have problems. My grandparents have told me that my whole life, I've always been 100% all in whether I was doing good things or bad things. So, if I did anything that got me in trouble, I was all in, and vice versa with things that were productive for me. And at that age, trouble was easy to find, and authority was more of a challenge for me now that I had so much independence.

A lot happened my senior year, including 9/11. The school put the videos of the planes hitting up in class and shortly after, everyone got released for the rest of the day. I remember feeling so horrible for the people who died and lost loved ones. It's still a vivid memory. It was not the reason I ended up joining the military, and honestly, I still have questions about 9/11: specifically about Building 7 and why the plane dropped at free-fall speed to the ground?

On September 13, just two days after the World Trade Center Towers were destroyed, I had an incident that pushed me back into isolation. There was a particular teacher who liked to give me a difficult time. She would point me out in class, make an example of me, and embarrass me. Her husband had committed suicide, and I felt she was using me as an outlet to get out her negative emotions. In hindsight I have compassion for her, but at the time it made me angry. One day I had enough of feeling spotlighted, and in front of the whole class I told her she was not allowed to talk to me anymore and she couldn't talk to me like that because my family wasn't going to allow it. I was being an insecure teenager and threatened her like

I was in the mafia or something. Nothing happened that day, but a couple days later, I ended up getting called to the principal's office.

I hadn't seen my dad in months, but he was there. I was shocked to see him. Usually when you get called to the office you have an idea of what you're in trouble for. But it had been several days since I had threatened the teacher so I didn't know she had reported the incident. I was surprised to see my father already in the principal's office when I opened her door. When I went in, I was told I was getting expelled.

The public school system can be a counterproductive environment for a lot of developing kids—especially anyone who has a different type of personality or learning style. Being a teacher requires EQ, and not all teachers have that much bandwidth. In public schools, if you're in an honors class you are more likely to have legitimate learning experiences, but if you are in regular classes, it can feel like county jail. Everyone talking, people throwing stuff; there is no order. Mine was an inner city, huge school. For all these reasons, I did not put a lot of stock or effort into school.

Now, I was being expelled for "terroristic threats." Since the 9/11 attack, all the codes for threats got elevated, and this got me expelled, which wouldn't have happened before the attacks. We had to get a lawyer and fight the school board over this. I was allowed back into school but ended up with in-school suspension. I spent most of my senior year in all-day detention and in a separate classroom from other students. I was isolated again. One of the things I really got into during this time was looking into Jim Morrison, the singer-songwriter for The Doors. It became an obsession. In many ways I was ready for another transformation before I graduated high school. But I was still figuring out how to do that.

When I was a senior in high school, I got to know another early mentor in my life, Johnny L., who was my girlfriend's father. When I lived at my grandparents' house while they were in Spain, I enjoyed having people over so I had nonstop parties. Always having people around gave me a sense of security from being alone in the house. I thought it was great until the neighbors complained and I got kicked out.

After getting kicked out of that house, I lived in the guest house at my girlfriend's place. I sat and talked with my girlfriend's father a lot. He was a successful businessman, but an alcoholic who loved to gamble. He didn't seem to get along with everybody, but he seemed to really get along with me.

He was a wealthy guy, and the main person he hung out with was a guy named Camel, who was the bookie in the town. And all these guys he dealt with were around when we hung out, too. He would tell me to walk into a room and connect with anyone. Whether it's a homeless guy or the most successful guy. Each person is just as important as the next person. And that's how I feel about life. You need to be able to walk with kings and be able to walk with people living on the streets. Everyone needs love and everyone matters.

Later in life I learned a poem by Rudyard Kipling that reminds me of some of the lessons I learned at this time, and it has helped some of the high-level athletes and executives I work with.

> If you can talk with crowds and keep your virtue,
>   Or walk with Kings—nor lose the common touch,
> If neither foes nor loving friends can hurt you,
>   If all men count with you, but none too much,
> If you can fill the unforgiving minute,
>   With sixty seconds' worth of distance run,
> Yours is the Earth and everything that's in it,
>   And—which is more—you'll be a Man, my son!

This has helped me to navigate life with more composure, self-control, integrity, and humility when the chips are up and when they are down as well. Anyone can pretend to be anyone they want when everything is smooth sailing. You find out who people around you really are when the ship is sinking. When the storm comes, you find out who is who within the circle of relationships you have in your life.

After an accomplished military career or when the championship belt is gone, and all the social media buzz is over, Ultimate Fighting Championship fighters, former champions, and sports icons across all domains experience a similar moment when all the smoke clears and their locker is cleared out. That moment could end up being years, decades, the rest of their lives as find their true selves now that their glory chapter has closed. To live in the present you must let go of attachment to these accomplishments in order to fully transition and allow new opportunities for present and future wins, feelings, and accomplishments.

CHAPTER 5

Treading Water

After high school, I received an academic scholarship to Texas Lutheran University, a private college in Texas. It made sense to go there because my Uncle Steve, someone I've always admired, had strong ties to the school. I went there for a couple of months, but from day one I didn't have an interest in being there. I saw a lot of students wearing tie-dye shirts and throwing frisbees and I didn't feel like I fit in or relate to anyone after my experiences up to this point. I tried to pretend for a little bit. I tried to go to classes but only went to a couple. My roommate was the dean's son, and he got expelled in the first semester. Nothing was going well so I ended up moving into an apartment off campus in San Antonio and enrolled at San Antonio Community College.

I also started working at this point and I had some crazy jobs.

I found a job at a telemarketing/tele-sales firm, selling mortgages and refinance packages for CitiFinancial. This was my first experience selling over a telephone and I treated it like a game. My job was to press a dial button, which would automatically call someone on my list to potentially sell to. If they did not own a home, then there was no point talking to them. That was the only disqualifier. If they did own a home, they were open game to convince them that they needed a new mortgage. If I got far enough to be able to transfer them to my manager, who would finish closing the sale, I would be compensated. I think I made $20–50 per call if I made a sale. This was a game and the experience taught me not to worry about rejection.

If I am going to make sales, I had to make a ton of calls and be willing to accept rejection if things don't align and create a win-win.

I also had paper routes and other odd jobs to make ends meet. I was even a live drawing model for a short while. This was a very interesting job, dropping my clothes in the middle of a room while people drew me for an hour at a time. This was a job that was scary at first but built confidence once I got the "hang" of it. (No pun intended.)

Eventually I quit school and left San Antonio. I moved in with my mom down near the border of Mexico and Texas. This is also when I started to work spring break seasonally at South Padre Island. This was typically one of the top three spring break destinations in the United States, so it was always wild and crazy times. Once spring break hits, it gets packed for two weeks straight, with different waves of parties, drinking, fights, drugs, crime, girls gone wild. Everything gone wild. I served drinks at the most popular resort. We had one guy and two girls serving drinks. I served all the females. Girls served the guys. There was a lot to keep me entertained and distracted and I started dabbling in different things.

Besides working the party scene, I also worked construction on the border of Mexico for my grandfather Papa's business. We would have these huge jobs with close to 100 people on the job sites. I learned a lot watching how my grandfather handled customers and a number of employees from rough backgrounds on these construction sites. Papa always set a positive and strong example for our family to follow and was looked at as the patriarch of the family.

Papa was an architect and he was well known in South Texas for his style of design; his inspiration came from Mexican Colonial architecture from the 1800s. I remember working on the job sites and having photographers come out to document the unique style.

My grandfather not only intentionally designed each feature of every house that he created but he also sourced a lot of the materials from a very special place in Mexico, San Miguel de Allende (St. Michael of legends). It was about a 12-hour drive one way from where we lived in South Texas to get down to San Miguel, and I loved to ride with my grandfather on those trips.

From when I was about 13, I was allowed to stay out in the *discotecas*, or discos, when we would go down to San Miguel, as it was pretty safe at that time for tourists. (I have not been there in 20 years so I cannot speak on what it is like there now.) At those clubs I was served alcohol and treated like a young adult. San Miguel was a destination for aspiring artists and there were always plenty of Americans down there to hang out with, as well as friendly locals. These experiences gave me a lot of street smarts and confidence to navigate the clubs and nightlife at a young age. I was cultured because my grandparents taught me and put me in situations where I had to figure things out, whether that be on the construction site or in the discos in Mexico.

My grandfather wasn't just building construction projects. He went out of his way to build me up, as he did all his grandchildren. I remember how much patience he had. It seemed like he was the most patient person in the whole world. I remember him getting his hand slammed in a truck door and not even flinching or complaining, and when he broke his arm when we were camping he didn't complain for one second.

My first trip to jail was while I was in Marine Military Academy (MMA) boarding school during high school. My friends and I would sometimes sneak past the academy's security guards and roving security vehicles to get off campus. We'd then walk to the airport that was down the street and access one of the vehicles one of us owned and kept off campus. Then we would go to South Padre Island or across the border to party in Mexico. Granted, most of my friends who were with us had some kind of political connections in Mexico, so they had no fear about navigating the streets, clubs, or Policia.

One night, one of the kids who was with us was so drunk he couldn't walk, and we ended up getting arrested coming back across the border. We spent the night in the jail and were released in the morning and return to MMA. We were all put on restriction for a little while, and I remember my grandfather dressed up really nice to come visit me after I got in trouble and was supportive, not judging me or being mad at me. He was very patient.

This happened more when I was arrested several more times. He was always the one to bail me out of jail. To be clear, my grandfather was hardcore with everyone on the job site. However, with me, he was always loving and kind. The last time I was in trouble and went to jail, he bailed me out and brought me home and cooked me a steak dinner. I will never forget something that he said to me that night: "When you make your first million dollars . . ." It refocused everything that night to how successful I would be one day in my life. I love my grandfather so much for everything he did for me, and most of the things I have accomplished in life have been because I wanted to make him and my Nana proud. I wanted to make my whole family proud, but especially them.

I learned a lot about life from seeing my grandfather operate as an architect. I did not come out with any of his skills in building design or mechanics, but I do believe that I am an architect with people. Investing in people, building alliances, and building connections that force multiply and support each other. I love that kind of building.

My grandfather always had a way of handling challenging people or situations. He gave me a lot of experience while watching him manage and deal with people who are hard to work with. Whenever he had to focus on another project, I would fill in on the job site. I got tested a lot because the other workers looked at me like I was the boss's son, and they wanted to see what, if anything, they could get away with. It made me resilient, and with practice I learned how to turn these relationships from obstacles into a win with mutual and long-term respect.

There were some positive things I gained from this time, but I did not feel a strong sense of purpose, so it was easy to get into things that were not healthy. There was a lot of crime and partying around me in my environment, and I started to spiral downhill. I got into partying, into drugs, and into trouble. I remember getting robbed a few times and I got into situations where I robbed somebody back. I ended up in jail a few times on either possession charges or public intoxication. When I worked as a bouncer at one point, I had a bunch of fake IDs and got in trouble for wrongful identification.

My anger issues were really starting to show, and I kept getting into more trouble. And again, my grandfather stepped in. I remember him picking me up from jail one of the times I got arrested. It was for an incident that was my biggest charge (but ended up getting dropped). I told him that I was just so grateful for him and getting me out of this situation and I wouldn't know what I would have done if he didn't support me.

There was a period when I started running, so he would take me every morning at 5 a.m. to the lake in town that had a track around it. I would run in one direction, and my grandfather would go in the other direction. And passing him every lap gave me strong motivation. I was balancing the lack of purpose on one hand and the drive to make my grandparents proud on the other hand.

Then one night I stayed up all night and waited for my grandfather to come out of his house for work. I stopped him and told him I was lost, and I didn't know what to do with my life.

He took in what I was saying and responded. "Remember when you went to Marine Military Academy and how much you liked it? Why don't we go talk to the marine recruiter."

At the time, I had *a lot* against me. A lot of legal cases and extra baggage weighing me down. So much that I didn't think enlisting would be a reality or even possible, but I was open to it. I was open to anything at this point, really. So, my grandfather took me to the recruiters where I did some testing. They took me to the Military Entrance Processing Station (MEPS) in San Antonio, where they took my fingerprints and looked at my background. When my record came back, it was like a rap sheet and the recruiter told me, "I'm sorry, this isn't going to work. We just don't see how we can work with all of this," and sent me on my way. I was very discouraged. All these breakdowns had taught me resilience, although it felt terrible at the time. Many of life's most terrible experiences can later become our biggest opportunities for breakthroughs.

A couple weeks later, a recruiter called me back and told me, "If you are willing to work through a process with us, we may have a chance of getting you a waiver." At the time I was ready, so I went in. And for every single arrest, ticket, or item on my record, I wrote statements for each one. And we got waivers for each incident. Anything we could possibly get to help make my case, we got. I had recommendations from three high-level officials and my drill instructor from military school. After about a year of going back and forth, completing paperwork, getting interviewed, and jumping through a lot of hoops, I finally got approval.

I know now that this was a special case. Because these days if you have *anything* on your record, it's almost impossible to get in the military. So, for me to have a significant amount on my record, including three drug charges, it was a miracle that I got in at all. And so I went to boot camp. If I had not gotten into the military, I cannot see how I would not have ended up in a penitentiary. I had been arrested five different times already. But getting through everything and enlisting into the marines was not an easy path.

My purpose and why was to make my family and grandparents proud. It carried me a long, long way through the hardest parts. Pretty much my entire military experience was fueled by making them proud.

Boot Camp

I was sent to San Diego for boot camp. I was blown away by the environment, atmosphere, and weather. Man . . . I thought this was a dream. Even little things, like looking at seagulls, were beautiful. The seagulls in San Diego were signals of abundance. The seagulls back in Texas looked like scavengers. They are savages. Like crows, they'll come in to snag your lunch if you set it on top of your car. They are like little fighters, but in San Diego they look like cartoons with these beautiful features.

Boot camp was easy for me. It was in downtown San Diego. They'd have us march for hours. We would march up a hill, look at crazy houses at the top, and the weather was incredible, especially coming from where I was from in Texas, where the heat and humidity can eat you alive. Everyone was just blown away by the weather, the environment, and views. Taking it all in was crazy.

It's important to note that the Marine Corps was founded in a bar, called Tun Tavern. And drinking has always been a huge part of the culture. And that's what I fell right into. I had come from South Padre Island, the type of area where there is nonstop partying. My extracurricular activities were partying, and I started out in trouble in the Marine Corps.

I was in the processing program for so long to get in, and I had to travel from where I lived to the processing station at MEPS. There were some marines at MEPS who had it out for me for creating friction and being there so many times. How I showed up or whatever I did always seemed to piss them off. This experience ultimately taught me to make friends, not enemies, with anyone who affects your professional career.

When you fly into California for boot camp, you wait in the United Service Organization facility inside of San Diego Airport and for the drill instructors to come pick you up. When we got there as a group, one of the drill instructors had been notified I was coming by somebody in San Antonio whom I had dealt with administratively at the MEPS there.

Immediately the drill instructor called for "Recruit Hall" to do push-ups. So, I saw how all of boot camp was going to be going ahead of time, before boot camp really even began. Right from the start, I pushed boundaries to see what this was really going to look like. I was looking for what their response would be whenever I could. What happens when I act tired, or don't listen, and just see what any of that did. I was testing to see what the environment was going to be. Are they going to kick me on the ground when I can't do more push-ups? I wanted to know what's actually going to happen.

Then started boot camp for everyone. The drill instructors would punish and make an example of me more than anyone else in the group. I seemed to welcome the hazing and special attention at times. These thrashings meant extended push-ups, jumping jacks, sit-ups, and planks for long periods of time, up to hours on one occasion.

I've always been very resistant to authority. At military boarding school, I loved my drill instructor there. He was a great mentor, a boxer, and overall great guy, and I respected him a lot. I surrender authority when I respect and trust the person. Great leaders command respect and poor leaders still try to *demand* respect. I knew I would resist when a poor leader demanded respect, and I stepped up to my fullest when I had a leader who commanded my respect through strong leadership and example.

I completed boot camp and my grandparents came to my graduation. It was almost a clean slate for me. They took me to Las Vegas for a few days of vacation. Then I went home for a few days before going to Infantry school at Camp Pendleton in California.

Infantry Combat Training

When I went into the marines, to get accepted I said I would take any job. They put me in as artillery because they needed those jobs filled, and I got into boot camp knowing that's where I'd be placed if I graduated.

I saw that all my friends in boot camp were going to infantry and into combat-type jobs. Artillery may do combat, but infantry are on the front lines. I wanted to be with my friends and do something that felt more important. In hindsight, I respect everyone's job specialty in the Marine Corps but this was my perspective and thought process at the time. I needed to figure out how to move from artillery into infantry. That was where my friends were going and where I wanted to go.

At the end of boot camp, we had about a week of administrative time to get in all our paperwork in order to go to our next training stop. This is where I started to make moves to get my MOS (military occupational specialty) changed from artillery to infantry. When I went home for vacation after boot camp, I thought I had done everything that I needed to officially go to the infantry course. However, when I got to Camp Pendleton, I was directed toward the line for the course that I did not want to be in. I was starting marine combat training. Despite the name, this was a 17-day crash course for all other jobs that were not war-fighter focused (cooks, administrative positions, etc.). The purpose was to give all these different types of marines with noncombat roles a taste of war fighting so that if they ended up deployed in a combat zone, they at least had a reference point for what a machine gun looks like, and how you might shoot it, for example.

The whole time during the training I was asking to switch. I didn't want to be there, I wanted to be in infantry training. Somebody was even asking for volunteers to move to infantry; I told every instructor that I wanted to go to infantry. Yet I was about to get permanently stuck doing the artillery job. A few days before graduating and being assigned to artillery school, I pulled the last stop that I had, which was to sit on my rack, aka bed (you are not allowed to ever sit on your rack in the marines and they are always supposed to be perfectly made), and tell the instructors that *I refuse to train*. Refusing to train was the same thing as calling a timeout. I said again I want to go to the infantry course; I don't want to graduate unless I get to go to the infantry course.

They ultimately said okay. I was given all new gear and got put into the infantry course.

In boot camp you don't get any time off base or free time, except one hour on Sundays. But in infantry school, we could go out on the weekends. We got into the pattern of going to San Diego, going to a hotel, taking a taxi, then a train, to San Diego State University sorority parties. For at least a month or two that was our weekend routine.

Sometimes we would go into the backyard of frat parties, set up some kind of diversion, while others would get some of the kegs and throw them over the fence. We'd then take a cab to the hotel and have our own party.

At one of those sorority parties, I noticed my wallet was gone. I started asking some of the frat guys who were there if anyone had seen it. Based on their responses, it seemed like they were in on something and did know. My wallet had my military ID, and I was stressed because I could not get on or off base without it.

Part of infantry school included enemy prisoner of war (EPW) training, which included wall searches (when you put someone's head against the wall, their arms behind their backs, lean their body against the wall, and search them) in preparation for deployment. They were teaching us how to do searches as safely as possible. So my buddies and I went through and did wall searches on everyone in the sorority house. But we didn't find my wallet. We later found out it had been left on the train and was with train security. I was able to get my military ID. It was all a misunderstanding and an alcohol-related incident.

That Monday morning after the party, we're all cleaning the bunk room. Our instructors started yelling for me and my buddy, whom I signed out with for the weekend. They were yelling at us like we were in trouble and to come to the office.

They put crime scene tape around my bed, lockers, and foot lockers. They had me sit outside on a bench all day, and made it seem and feel like I was under arrest in the military. I sat on this bench, while all these guys I was in infantry school with for three months had to give a written statement.

It seemed like some of my friends were switching sides on me about what happened that weekend during their interrogations by the instructors. The frat guys wanted to get some revenge, I guess for embarrassing them at the party. One of the guys from the party got my name and said that I was selling drugs at the party. It wasn't true, I didn't have any drugs, and luckily, I wasn't involved in any of that.

I got pulled out of training and anyone who had seen me that weekend was interviewed. They all had different perspectives. They thought they would get in trouble, so I ended up just sticking with my story. I wasn't going to snitch on myself for something I didn't do. I took a drug test and went back to training. I could have easily been kicked out of the marines with this incident.

After barely graduating infantry school due to my extracurricular actions, I was sent to my first duty station at beautiful Camp Pendleton, California. When I got to my first unit, I ended up in a sniper unit. Sniper training was a series of constant tests, similar to how mentally and physically tough some of the special operations training would be.

Our sniper commander liked to test us, and it felt like he was playing games with everyone who had not been to sniper school yet (even though he had not been to sniper school himself). Sometimes he went too far. One day I got the horrible news that my stepmom had died. I received a Red Cross message, and my commander and other leadership informed me to make arrangements to fly home to Texas, which I immediately did. I dressed and was about to leave when our sniper commander said, "I'm sorry, these things happen, but I need you to get changed; you're not going to be able to go home." Not being able to get on the plane and go to my stepmom's funeral flipped a switch in me. I was now against everyone who was there, and I ended up having the worst performance. I didn't want to do anything. I wanted to sabotage everyone who was involved. Playing those kinds of games was not acceptable to me. I had a lot of anger because of this situation. I ended up getting kicked out of a sniper platoon and got put into a regular infantry company. I can look back now and see how all the trauma and authority issues compounded for the worse. My experience with the sniper platoon was a huge motivation to pass my Marine Raider tryouts. This was another example of a painful challenge that ultimately launched me into success.

In military culture, there are some people in charge of other people only because they have a higher rank and a culture of yelling. So when I would drink, anyone I had any grievances with would easily trigger me. If somebody gave an order during the day that I thought was bullshit, or something disrespectful occurred, then at night I wanted to go find that person and flip the script. I was in flux going between Dr. Jekyll and Mr. Hyde. Any amount of alcohol was a recipe for chaos and a lack of discipline and self-control.

I ended up getting into two major alcohol-related incidents where I disrespected a staff officer and physically put hands on somebody who was a much higher rank than I was. I had no rank on my collar because I was constantly in trouble. I'd get promoted, then get knocked back down to private. It was during this time that I was introduced to Blackjack Matthews, who was invited to speak to our unit shortly before we deployed.

Lt. Colonel Blackjack Matthews was the officer in charge of the Beirut Barracks in Lebanon that turned over command three months prior to the 1983 bombing when 231 marines were killed. He had all these issues drinking, and when he told his story, I related so much. Like him, I had experiences of blacking out, not remembering anything that happened the night before. Like most young marines, if I had to go hear a speaker like this, I tended to just go in and kind of check out/daydream. But this guy really won me over.

I'd had the same rank of private or private first class for three years. I was always in trouble. A lot of it was because I had so much trauma from childhood that I hadn't self-regulated or processed. I didn't know how to separate those issues from the issues I was having in the Marine Corps.

In 2007, barely on my first deployment, I had been on restriction off and on for about a year and was working on making a comeback when I had a huge relapse and alcohol-related incident in Okinawa. And this time it was worse. The situation was crazy and afterwards, it was like somebody else entirely was there, not me. I have no memory of it. And it was a big deal because the person I got into an altercation with was a much higher rank. This caused a lot of trouble for me, and I almost got kicked out. But that was it for me and drinking.

Learning to Manifest

During this time, my grandmother was trying to teach me to understand the concept of manifestation, and she sent me a copy of the book *The Secret*. What I ultimately took away from this book was the practice of setting intention. When I decided to quit drinking was when I learned how to manifest a new reality for myself. And I started to live with intentionality, embrace experiences, and begin integration (especially as I got more clear from not consuming alcohol and adding lots of exercise into my life). And that's what I do every morning to this day. I set an intention for the day, go through my day and integrate that intention. Setting intention helps unlock your greatest potential. Your intention drives everything. And with practice you see patterns. You set an intention, go on a journey, then you must integrate it at the end of the day. That's the flow. And I've learned that the same pattern applies to healing, and when applied with that purpose, it can unlock powerful results. Every day and time you set a new intention and integrate it, you're building this practice for yourself.

After I made the decision and set the intention that I wasn't going to drink any more, I started training my ass off and working my way back up. This is when I got into the physical and mental shape I needed to progress. I was not in the mental shape to go into special operations while drinking and never would be. I went 10 years without drinking, from July 2007 until 2017.

CHAPTER 6

Marine Raiders, Gung Ho

Preparing for Selection

When I say I started training my ass off, I put *all* my effort, energy, and focus into it. I was running, swimming, and rucking (moving long distances with a weighted pack). And I was working with a mental focus trainer who would train me sometimes 6–10 hours a day, three-plus days a week. I would do my Marine Corps training, then go work extra with my trainer for hours. My performance at work went through the roof. I caught back up with my peers with rank because I started getting meritorious promotions and piling them up.

I was finally feeling good about myself. In my second deployment I reached four years of being in the military, which was the length of my original contract. I was taking it one enlistment at a time. At the end of my second deployment, at the end of four years, I had a package to go to special operations training, but to move forward, I needed to reenlist to have enough time on my contract to do that.

But my reenlistment was denied. I had too many alcohol-related incidents on my record. I had enough to result in multiple nonjudicial punishments and rank losses. My commander didn't want to approve me. In the Marine Corps, you're not supposed to go outside the chain of command. You don't plead your case directly; it must go up the system the proper way.

But there was a high-ranking enlisted marine, one of my old superiors, who knew my history and who worked alongside the commander. I caught him on the street at Al Asad Air Base during my last week in Iraq.

"Excuse me, Sergeant Major," I said, "Please look at me. Do you remember me? I used to always be in trouble and lost my rank." I pled my case. Told him I'd stopped drinking, explained how much I'd grown, and that I was a different person now. I told him I had a package ready for special ops, if I could just get reenlisted.

He went to bat for me. And I got approved.

I reenlisted and headed to selection in North Carolina, a month-long assessment where I met Don Tran, who would go on to become one of my closest friends, business partner, and cofounder of Deep End Fitness (DEF) and Underwater Torpedo League (UTL).

I'm grateful that I started out in the infantry. I hit a lot of peaks and valleys during this time. There were so many moments I was in a dark place, and in so much trouble, I even lost rank twice. It came to a point where I had enough failures that I was at the risk of being kicked out. My quality of life wasn't great.

While I was in the infantry most of my time was spent as a machine gunner. This meant that during training or deployment, I was always carrying a machine gun and a heavy pack. The mental and physical rigor it demanded gave me a strong baseline and it set me up for success in special operations.

In the infantry, everything is conventional. You're conditioned to operate inside a box. But what I know about myself is that I don't perform well when I feel boxed in or constrained. When I'm outside the box, or when there's no box at all, my performance skyrockets. That's when I can improvise, innovate, and adapt. That's when I find meaning and purpose.

The rigid structure of the infantry, combined with my natural resistance to authority, fueled me to not go back into infantry. I was deeply motivated to get out, make it through selection, and earn my place in special operations as a Marine Raider. At the time, the unit was called MARSOC, which stood for Marine Special Operations Command. In 2016, we were officially renamed Raiders again, which helped solidify our identity within USSOCOM (United States Special Operations Command).

My first deployment was extended from six months to a full year-long trip across the Pacific. It was grueling. In that deployment, we flew to Okinawa, Japan, got on a ship, and went to South Korea where we dug holes in the middle of wintertime. We went back to Australia and did a month-long patrol in the rainforest, 30 days nonstop patrolling, sleeping only a few hours a night, and moving all day long. A lot of people broke and mentally snapped. From there we went to the Philippines, where we lived in the fields for a month and trained with the Philippine marines, and then back to Okinawa. We experienced no combat in this deployment, but everyone still talked about it.

In 2008 I was sent on a deployment to Iraq. The biggest thing that stood out to me about this period was how much all the marines who were senior to me—who had been there before—were talking about combat all the time. So, combat was what I prepared myself for.

When we went to Iraq, there was not much combat. There were some indirect fire, some rockets that would come into the base, some improvised explosive device (IEDs), some bombs and bomb threats, but it was not some crazy combat zone like it had been in the years before. This was because the United States was transitioning everything over to the Iraqis at this time.

So, this really felt like another training deployment. This one was a pretty miserable experience for me. I didn't like being in the conventional military at all, where you must blindly follow rules and orders, just because this is how it's always been done, or this is how we do it.

All these more senior guys were talking about being deployed and in combat. They had been there and done that and talked about it like it was a rite of passage, part of the club that you could only have access to if you had been in combat. I would later find out, once I was living in the reality of it, to be careful what you wish for. You really know once you are there. In Afghanistan the enemy knew exactly where we were at and living because we were living in an enemy village. That village was where we were at, engaging with the local police, and being attacked almost every day. We were protecting ourselves and dealing with the situation the best that we could. Once I was out of this experience entirely, I just wanted peace. My cage was rattled to say the least. I never wanted to deal with these types of experiences again. I would never want anyone I cared about to go through something like this.

After this deployment and my reenlistment, I was waiting to go to selection for special operations. Selection is essentially a one-month tryout of assessment and selection. At Camp Pendleton there was a pool called Camp Horno Pool. This was a great training pool where a lot of combat marines trained. This was the most active out of any pools on base at the time. This was a huge win for me. I was fortunate to get to work there as my job while I was training for selection. This meant that my main job was to train and get ready and spend a few hours a day training marines in water confidence. Compared to my infantry unit where I had to be available 24/7—*this was a win!*

There were a few marines who helped me get the job at the pool, Alex Queen and Harry Majszak. Queen put me through my initial tests to get the job and then I was sent to Marine Corps Instructor of Water Survival (MCIWS) course. I had absolutely no idea at the time, but my experience at the pool working as a water survival instructor would be a critical skill that I would end up using in multiple ways, especially after the Marine Corps in the work we do with DEF and UTL.

While I was there, I wanted to get feedback from anyone who had been out for selection. I wanted to learn why people fail or quit. I was learning that a lot of it had to do with the pool, and people were failing because of the water. This happened not just in selection but also in the 10-month individual training course (ITC) that happens after selection.

I trained all the time; I got to the pool and focused. I went to a three-week MCIWS course to get more proficient because I hadn't spent a lot of time in the pool during my time in the infantry. But I had grown up swimming in a pool. I lived near the ocean the whole time growing up in Texas, so I loved the water and I loved working at the pool in Corpus Christi. It was my favorite job in the Marine Corps, too.

The MCIWS course was very challenging because I sink like a rock in water. It was challenging to swim the amount we did, tread water all day, swim with all the gear, do rescues and other exercises. But after the course, I went back to the pool and started getting repetitions as an instructor and training marines who would come through for their annual training. I had no idea at the time how this experience laid the foundation for what I do today.

Water training gives us a special access: a window into our soul and a look inside of ourselves where we can lean in and improve or even shift something that might not be working for us. Once we have more awareness over our mind and limitations, we can start to take action to create small wins. As we stack those wins, we create more flow and confidence to set boundaries and eliminate drag in different areas of life.

Selection

Right before leaving for selection, I went home to Texas to spend time with my grandparents and get my mind ready for the next chapter of my life.

While I was home, I was informed that my great uncle, who had been a marine during the Korean War, wanted to speak to me before I went into Marine Raider training. When I called him, I was surprised when he told me that he served with Marine Raiders and that it was not going to be a good fit for me, that I should look into doing something else besides special operations in the marines.

This really angered me, but it was a blessing in disguise. I would remember this conversation in the coming years when I needed a little "push" in training. I would think about what my uncle told me and how I was proving him wrong. It gave me an extra gear to shift into when I needed to show up and perform at a higher level.

In hindsight, I don't think my uncle really knew what he was talking about, but it is a lesson in life for when people doubt you and try to project their own limitations and fears onto you. If you ever experience this type of behavior, *do not let it hold you back for one second*. Use it as fuel to break through to the next levels of life.

When I went to the special operations assessment and selection course, I met Don Tran at one of the very first training events. You're not really allowed to talk to anyone unless you are working with them, and even then, you are being evaluated the whole time. Don and I connected at that event, helped each other, and from then on it's become our history.

We both got selected after a month and went back to Camp Pendleton. We knew we were going to the ITC, and we worked it out that Don and our other buddy, Andrew (aka Camp), could come to work at the pool, so the three of us started working and training together at the pool. We focused on getting ready for the ITC for a good 6–9 months.

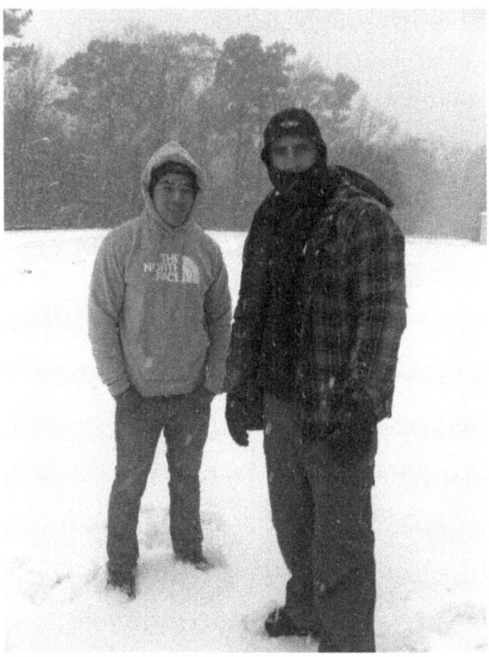

Prime with Don Tran at ITC Raider Training
in North Carolina (2011)

To get ready we were lucky enough to have full access and full rein of the pool. We also had an outdoor gym at the pool that we called *Muscle Beach*, which consisted of a bunch of rusted weights on the side of the pool, that we loved to train with. We used the weights above water and underwater, working with the torpedoes, running the hills of Camp Pendleton, and going on pack runs. We worked and prepared nonstop. On top of that we were training marines who were coming back for their annual training, so we were also getting thousands of repetitions in of instruction with water confidence. If you can train somebody to swim for the first time or to have a breakthrough in the pool, it can also teach you a lot about unlocking results and breaking through fear. We didn't realize then how valuable that experience was, how it would play out later, and how we would use it in real life. But this set us up and put us on a trajectory for future success.

When we got to the ITC in North Carolina, every Wednesday we had pool days. Each week at 5 a.m. we would ride the bus to the pool. The atmosphere was always gloomy; nobody wanted to go. The way they ran these sessions put most students into fight-or-flight mode. We had to do a lot of underwater challenges like tying knots or other things that people weren't very comfortable doing. Most didn't have the water confidence or foundation to deal with the challenges that were given to us at the pool on Wednesday mornings. Don, Camp, and I did great in the water because we had been training so much. We were comfortable and relaxed. Of course, we had challenges as well, but we stayed connected, worked together, did our thing, and helped our teammates as much as possible in the water.

On the flip side, after about a day or two I realized I was one of the slowest runners in the whole pack. Just imagine coming from being a conventional unit in the Marine Corps, where I was one of the fastest, to going the special ops unit, where I was one of the slowest guys. On the runs, I felt like I was drowning. However, in the pool I was faster than most and could tread for long periods of time and had a decent breath hold. I remember how much I needed the small victories in the pool to carry me through some of the losses I was taking on the long runs we did every morning. It was hard to adjust at first but ended up being a huge gift and lesson to never give up when you feel like you suck, because even if you are weak in one area, you can always make up and overcome it on the next event or challenge.

It was an opportunity to learn and accept that I will not always be great at something and to learn to take losses. I discovered how to show up for my team in other ways to still add value. For instance, my team had to deal with me sucking at runs. How could I add value in other ways so that I was carrying my weight with the team? I knew I could contribute at the pool with training and adding water confidence to the guys, as well as helping with anything else I could think of, like boosting morale, telling jokes, taking one for the team. These were the things I learned to do. I sucked on the runs, which bothered me, but I'm grateful looking back because I learned emotional intelligence. I'm grateful because if I was the fastest, the number one runner, I might not have found other ways to find value or open the door for the relationships I had with the guys around me.

Don Tran, Camp, and I ended up on the same team together the whole time at ITC. We were there for each other as a reinforced buddy system, and that was such a blessing. There were times when my mind shut off, especially when it was due to sleep deprivation, or in the hell week, aka Raider Spirit, an intense two-week field exercise with little to no sleep. I would be there physically, but my mind shut off. This is when Camp or Don or other team members would help carry me or push me until I came alive again. We all supported each other during these hallucinations and periods of mindlessness.

Camp recently visited me in San Diego and reminded me of a time that he had to carry me on his shoulders down a mile-long road during one night of our hell week training. It is a reminder to me of how important it is to have a support system around you, especially during challenging times.

I learned in my first two deployments how important it is to have one solid buddy and, depending on how capable your buddy is, that can make or break you. Having that support system was completely outside of my comfort zone, besides the experience I had with using the buddy system on my first and second deployment. But in these times of not eating or sleeping for several days, carrying heavy weight for days without any sleep, dealing with hallucinations in the middle of the woods, I don't see how you can make it through alone without a support system around you. You can't do these things by yourself. Not everyone got through ITC. Our class dropped so many people.

I'm grateful for Don, Camp, and all the badass teammates we had in our ITC Class (Class 1-11). They are what got me through.

After we got through S.E.R.E. (survive, evade, resist, escape) training; amphibious training in Key West, Florida; and Raider Spirit, we finally moved on to the shooting phase. One day, we had to go during the lunch break to do a fast rope simulation, where you slide rope in preparation for a real drop out of a helicopter at night, which we were going to do a few days later. For this simulation, we had to go to a training tower, in full gear, and do fast rope slide drills. You had to throw the fast rope gloves on, slide down the rope, climb back up a tall staircase to get back to the top of the rope, and repeat.

On the last repetition, I performed a parachute landing fall, the standard way to land when jumping out of an aircraft. I landed, rolled, and got up to rejoin the team. Then I heard the instructors:

"No. Get back."
"Do it again."
"Again."
"Again."

They had me repeat this procedure over and over again.

My teammates went back to the shooting house. I stayed at the training tower for a few hours with the instructors who were trying to see if they could break me. Or maybe they were trying to test me to see if they could ultimately trust me. I had seen this happen to different students since training began. When it happened to me, we were probably seven months or more into training. I was past the point of no return. Really, day one is the point of no return if you're going to make it through.

Getting singled out by the instructors is a make-or-break moment. It's sink or swim. If you fuck it up when the heat's on, you'll get dropped from the course. By that point, we'd seen plenty of classmates dropped for all kinds of reasons—some seemed warranted, some not. Everyone was on edge. If you failed here, it could become the story of your life.

So, there I was—my team gone, and just the instructors left. All of them. Playing games, making me repeat the rope drill over and over.

"Again."
"Again."
"Again."

Something flipped in my mind. I snapped back into that mental focus training I'd done with my old trainer. He used to make me hold a stick out for hours until I shook. And when he'd finally say, "You're done," I'd look at him and say, "Fuck you. You're done."

I locked into that hyper-focused zone. I told myself, *These instructors are stuck here with me, too. And I'm prepared to go all day.*

I didn't ask for mercy. Didn't even look at them. Just hit the ground, got up, and did it again.

And again.

And again.

After an hour or two of this, I had another hard landing. I got up, rolled out, and was heading back up when they stopped me, saying, "You're done. Take off your gear and go sit in the bleachers."

I could tell they were trying to play it off as a safety violation and were looking for a way to drop me from the course. So, I stood next to the wall with all my gear still on.

"Get your gear off," they said again, "You're done."

"No," I replied, "I'm not done. I can do this all day."

"Oh really . . . ," they said, and they made me prove it.

They threw me back on the rope. Again. And again. This repeated all afternoon.

I drew on every ounce of resilience I had. They tested me to see if I could endure the impossible. To see if I could be trusted to go beyond what was expected.

Then they put me on the 90-foot rope and had me doing lockouts. That's where you slide down at full speed, then stop instantly when they yell, "Lockout!"

You freeze right where you are on the rope. No hesitation. They kept playing those games, but I made it through, rejoined my team, and finished out the day.

It wasn't until the next morning at the gym that I realized something was wrong. I tried to bench press 135 pounds just to warm up, but my arms were shaking. I couldn't even move the weight. Then I tried just the bar. Same thing, my arms were shaking and I couldn't move the weight. It turned out, both of my biceps were torn.

My biceps were super painful then. Even now, if I overtrain or the weather shifts fast, I feel it flare up with a sharp, lingering pain. The pain in my biceps is nothing compared to the pain I would have had if I had been dropped at the end of ITC.

As we approached the final week of the shooting training, we prepared for our final qualifications on the range and inside the shoot house. This was where we run through and shoot in the house, with live ammunition. They set up all your magazines with different malfunctions and problems.

But I didn't give a flying f*ck about any of the malfunctions because my arm was so shaky. I got through it; they thought I was nervous, and maybe I was, but the bigger issue was that my bicep was ripped. Regardless, I finished it.

In the final stage of the qualification phase, I called out one of the instructors. The thing is, once I called them out, they were accountable, an illusion shattered in my mind, and it felt like watching a house of cards fall. I couldn't have done it in the middle of training because they would have set me up, saying I did something unsafe, and fail me. However, once we were done with all that training and ready to move onto the next phase, I was able to say what I needed to say—how fucked up they were and how they mistreated students. To their credit, the Marine Raiders school was fairly new at that point, and it didn't have a good foundation on how to operate as instructors yet. Another credit to them is that the bullshit they put us through and stress from that experience makes most areas of life feel pretty easy after you make it through. Today, I am grateful for all of them and for the experience. At the end of the day, they did their job and we were prepared.

After the qualification phase, we had about a month or two left of training before graduating Luckily, I got sent back to Camp Pendleton, to the 1st Marine Special Operations Battalion (1MSOB).

Don, Camp, and I were stationed together along with Derek Herrera and Ricky Briere. Most of us were super happy about going back to California because we were West Coast marines to begin with and we didn't want to be stuck in the swampy area in North Carolina. We wanted to get back to California fast. I can still vividly remember getting back, looking around, and enjoying the scenery. I was so grateful to be back in this amazing place.

I had one girlfriend during this time in the marines. We were long distance the whole time during the special operations training, and we had problems and fought nonstop. She was supposed to meet me in California when I moved back but the word that I was getting from the unit was that I needed to be ready to deploy to Afghanistan right after we returned. I ended up breaking up with my girlfriend. I wanted to cut away from the drag and focus on what I had in front of me. So when I got back to California, I was single, focused, and ready to work.

Every Day Is a Tryout

Imagine going through a 10-month course, where you are being evaluated the entire time, and it's the hardest thing you've ever done in your life. You did all these different things to get through it successfully. Then you get to your unit where nobody knows anything about what you did because it was a new thing. Nobody gives a f*ck about what you did or has a reference point for it. Crazy enough, that ended up being a huge positive that forced us to show up in our new unit and earn our spot every day. It taught and reinforced to me that it doesn't matter what you did yesterday; it matters what you bring to the table today. That is a good lesson.

Nobody wants to listen to the guy who just talks about what he was doing back in the day and who is not making any moves to grow, improve, or evolve. You are always being evaluated. There was a saying in my unit: "Every day is a tryout." And it really was. Especially for a new guy. You have to prove yourself. I had been to Iraq, but I didn't have a lot of actual combat experience. I didn't have a lot of different skill sets and hadn't been to any advanced schools at that time like everyone else. Everyone in our unit was so experienced and could add value to the team in a second. As a new guy, I didn't have all that yet, but I got put on my first team and I started to operate and actuate what I had been training for all these years. The stakes were very high, and we all felt it in different ways. This seemed like the pinnacle of modern warfare for the Marine Corps, and it was a very fast-paced environment that bred innovation and performance at the highest levels.

One of the things I loved most about being in special operations was the meritocracy. If you are a high performer or have a solution for something, you have input. Rank is secondary to performance.

You accept it and start to thrive every day instead of resisting the requirement of showing up and proving yourself every day. You begin to shift your mindset into welcoming new tryouts and embrace the fact that you are being tested, evaluated, and challenged. You can prepare yourself as best as possible to be ready when those times come. Once you're through the challenge, you can learn from it, debrief from it, and get better.

Preparing for Afghanistan

My captain, Derek Herrera, was my first Marine Raider team leader. He's had a huge impact on me. He is one of my closest friends and a mentor to me to this day. Derek pulled me onto his team, and we started training for Afghanistan for our first deployment together. I remember the first time he brought me in for my first review and we talked about my goals. I explained I wanted to add value to the team, but I wasn't sure how as the new guy. He put me as the armorer, which meant I helped manage all the gear, weapons, and equipment for the team. That was how I started out and I really loved it. It was cool, as the new guy, to be managing all these weapons. I had an amazing experience doing this. In a role like that you must work hard. You must maintain and hold accountability for every piece of equipment. You cannot lose or misplace one piece of serialized equipment or people could get fired from their job. Every item must be accounted for multiple times every month, and before and after every training operation.

We spent several months with our team and the other Raider teams that would be deploying with us to Afghanistan, getting ready and building cohesiveness. There were very few new guys on the team. The memories I have of all of us training back then are amazing. This was exciting time, a proving ground and a huge opportunity to learn from the senior leadership who had had multiple combat deployments as Raiders.

At the very end of our training work-up, before we went to Afghanistan, we got another team member. Ricky Briere. Ricky is also one of the most important people in my life. He is one of the biggest driving forces and best instructors for DEF and UTL. He had been at ITC but we had been on different teams.

Before the whole team deployed, I was sent in advance to take accountability of all our weapons and equipment. Another part of my job was to work with local Afghan police to plan training and missions to support the security of the area.

We were going to an enemy village in Helmand Valley, Afghanistan, and we were going to be there for seven months. The news that we were getting on the team already there was pretty crazy, as they were facing with enemy combatants. Once winter ends and the weather starts to heat up, the combatants flip (sell) the poppy (used to make opium, heroin, and opioids) and get money for weapons and ammo. Then they fight all summer long until it gets cold again.

Puppy Mission Rescue

Being a water person, I was fortunate to have a canal right in front of the compound during my Afghanistan deployment. With temperatures reaching 130°F and no showers available, the canal became my refuge. I could jump in to cool off and even shampoo my hair. It was a huge win in such harsh conditions. Of course, it wasn't ideal. It wasn't the cleanest body of water. Once I spotted a huge dead cow floating in the water. That killed the vibe for a few days to want to jump in. Even with that, having the canal nearby in Nahr-e-Saraj was one of the best things about being there.

A few weeks into my time there, the local Afghan police gifted me a couple of pigeons. These birds had weights around their feet, which kept them from flying away, so they just hung around. Not long after, they brought me another gift: a puppy named Naree. It was an Afghan Shepherd, or a Kuchi dog.

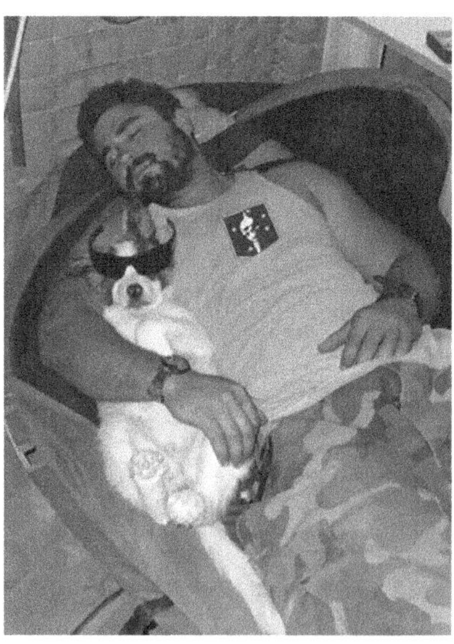

Prime with His Dog Naree in Helmand Valley (2012)

Having a dog was a special experience. I took care of her the best I could with what we had. Eventually, I was able to get proper food for her. About five months into the deployment, I reached out to the Puppy Rescue Mission. Thanks to donations, they arranged for her transport to Kabul and onward to my aunt and uncle's house in Texas, which was near an airport. She lived with them for almost 12 years. Every time a plane flew overhead, she would get low to the ground, almost as if she was hiding from an airstrike. Those instincts stayed with her. Naree passed away in 2024, but her story and her resilience remain a bright spot.

Afghanistan Quicksand

There were some crazy things that happened in this deployment. I saw things in Afghanistan I could have never dreamed of seeing in Iraq, such as people popping out of the ground from underground tunnel systems. It was mind blowing. One of the wildest things I saw was when our team ran into a quicksand-like mud pit situation. We had been setting up a fighting position in the village at night, and the buildings we went to occupy were saturated with bombs placed around the building and entry ways, so we had to go over the walls. But the walls to these buildings were too tall for us to get over with our equipment. We had to find an alternate building to occupy, but there was only one problem: the sun was coming up. We knew that the Taliban would surround us as soon as the daylight hit if we were still in the open field. We needed to act fast, but as we were moving toward the new compound, we ran into a huge mud pool that started to sink as we went through it. Most of our team and Afghan partners ended up stuck and could not move at certain points.

We were stuck like molasses there, and had to pull each other, wiggle, and dig ourselves out of that thing to get to the other side.

I remember some of our Afghan partners were trying to use their weapons in the mud, like a cane, and then they tried to pull themselves out. People were almost trying to fight each other to get up. For a while it felt like we were not going to get out. We didn't know where this stretch of mud started or ended. We were stuck with our heavy packs, trying to keep our weapons out of the mud. We ended up making it out, as a group; we would help if one person got stuck and we started to move quickly.

Makin' It Happen

We had arrived in Afghanistan in March just as it was starting to heat up. The base had already been attacked a couple times before we got there. Nothing major yet, just little attacks. It started getting us in the mindset and started to build urgency about the seriousness of the situation. Our base was located in the middle of an enemy village. We were surrounded on all sides, with problems to solve and obstacles to deal with, literally everywhere, for seven months.

If you went out during the day, you would get shot at. If you poked your head above the wall during the daytime, the Taliban would send a couple of rounds your way. They were watching you at *all* times. It was a real deal, 360-degree modern warfare situation. Often when we were attacked, there would be a couple grenades shot at us, by way of underbarrel grenade launchers multiple times a day at very close range.

Our team had a motto that one of our senior guys came up with. Before we deployed, we all got muscle shirts made with our team logo on the front and on the back: "Makin' it happen." This is still to this day one of my mottos in life.

Our team was in a situation that almost seemed impossible to deal with for seven months. We did it though. We did it as a team. We went through every emotion that a person has. We had laughs, cries, and everything else. We made it happen. We had a lot of wounded men on the team, but we didn't lose one guy. There were a ton of deaths that happened in general during that deployment, between our counterparts, the Afghans, or the enemy, but none for our team. I'm grateful for that—I was also very saddened and deeply affected by the deaths of the Marine Raiders on other teams who were killed in action while we were there.

Unsung Heroes

During that deployment, pretty much something happened every day, and there were a couple of major events. When we were just over a month into it, we went on a mission to a village to support an

TASK & PURPOSE

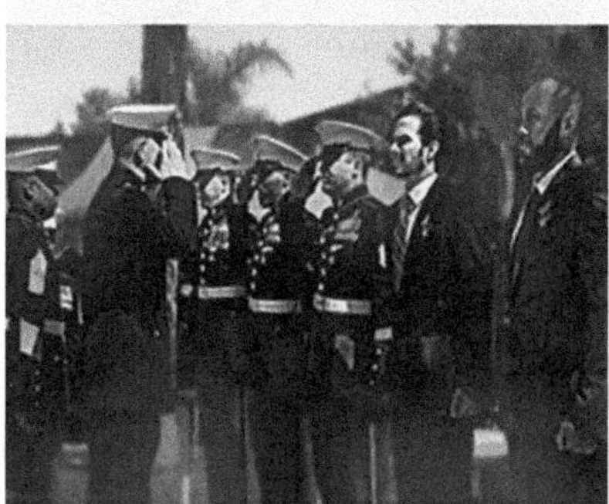

UNSUNG HEROES:
Surrounded And
Outnumbered, This MARSOC
Team Endured Hell To
Evacuate Their Wounded

Article Published in "Task and
Purpose" About the Events of
June 14, 2012

army special forces team with an operation they had going on. We got into a village in the middle of the night that we hadn't been to before. We got to the building and took it over, staying up all night, reinforcing the building, filling sandbags, figuring out how we were going to set up security and how we were going to fight our way out of this building for the next day. We were picking out holes in the compound where we could shoot from if or when we needed to, and also scanning the area for security with our night vision.

By the time it was 3:00 or 4:00 or in the morning, before the sun came up there was reporting of enemy activity and we knew we needed to set up another position for our team. We needed to take part of the team and get them out of the building toward a nearby tree line so that we could have two positions that we could mutually support each other in case one got overrun. So, a small group of guys and I went to the tree line a few hundred meters away with some of our Afghans and interpreters. We brought only our weapons, ammo, and whatever water we had on us.

As the sun was coming up, and shortly after we heard the sounds from the call to prayer, we could see people poking out their heads and looking at us from pretty much every area of this village. They were sneaking around, running from place to place, and their demeanor was very alarming. We knew things were about to be very intense. You could just feel that the whole world was about to drop. Our senses were on high alert. Full spidey senses. For me, I can remember thinking, *What the f*ck is happening?* I had a machine gun at the time, and we were in an area filled with IEDs, and the ground was saturated with little and big mines. If you stepped on one, it's your last step. You'll either die or lose your legs, or the guy behind you will lose his legs or maybe his face.

Every step that you take or any time that you lay down, or take a knee, you must be very diligent and process the area before you take a step or do anything. It's a full minefield everywhere because we were actually in a bomb-making village. There were IEDs and bombs everywhere. That was something that limited us from being able move quickly because we had to process this while minesweeping. Literally everywhere, people were getting blown up all day long. Every day we would hear explosions going off around us as well as in the distance.

As the morning started, there was an enemy running outside the compound that our team was in and trying to run into it. Several of the enemy got shot by our teammates, but once they were shot, the enemy knew where our team was. Once that happened a hail of enemy gunfire came into the room in the compound and on the fighting position we had built on the roof that was occupied by our team commander Derek and teammate Ricky.

Derek and Ricky were both shot and wounded on the rooftop. They were shot within five seconds of each other. We heard Derek come over the radio calling in that he's been wounded, and he needed help and a medic. He was so clear and calm on the radio, "I'm hit . . . ." It still blows my mind; I don't know how he was so clear because when he was shot, he was paralyzed from the chest down.

The medic was right next to me, an amazing person and teammate named Jordan, aka Ginger. When we heard Derek over the radio, teammates Will and Feez immediately started bounding back to the compound. Everyone who was with us jumped up from the tree line and started running back to the compound to support Ricky and Derek. Ginger and I ran together, but it took me a moment to get running. He waited for me as I worked to pull my pack on. My pack had all the machine gun ammo and once it was on, I still needed to reach down and grab the machine gun before I could take off. As we were running, we were engulfed by enemy fire. If you hear snaps and it seems that the ground is snapping around you, it means that the fire is *very* close. It's effective. This moment was one of the closest calls I've ever had in my life.

In that moment, it was all snaps of machine gun fire and whatever else they were shooting at us. Everything seemed to move in slow motion the whole time we were running back to the compound. Ginger was a faster runner than me, and I remember yelling at him to run faster, but we couldn't. It felt like time morphed into slow motion. Ginger was doing somersaults. Rolling and flipping and getting back up to keep running. I kept thinking he was falling from getting shot, but he was just dropping down and rolling.

When we got back to the compound, we checked ourselves, completely out of breath, but we were able to confirm we hadn't been shot, which was a miracle. Then we went in and heard the situation. Ginger's a medic, so he went in first and started working with the other guys who were saving Derek and Ricky.

Derek and Ricky were both in critical condition. Our teammates and medics who worked on them did miracle work, basically God's work. Our teammate Brian Jacklin, aka Jack, had taken charge in the middle of the situation and was recognized and awarded with a Navy Cross for his actions that day, the second highest valor of war in the military, just under a medal of honor. Jacklin had been in charge of me since I joined the team a year before. He mentored me and prepared all of us as much as possible. He seemed to be born for moments like that one when all hell broke loose that morning of June 14.

Afghan President Karzai has passed a law right before this that said that no more bombs would be dropped in the villages by the American military during combat operations. But we were in a situation where we had two marines critically wounded, in an enemy village before 7 a.m., and we were fully surrounded by enemy fighters who were going to completely overrun and destroy us. We needed the authority to drop bombs. Thankfully Jack had the initiative and the ability, confidence, and action in himself to call on the satellite phone and talk to the commanders to get authority to drop bombs. Had he not done that, we would not have survived. Had everyone on the team—Will, Feez, Dave, Chris, Ryan, and all our teammates and Afghan counterparts who rose to the occasion— not shown up in those moments, we would not have survived.

From there, we had a very small window of time to get the guys on the helicopters to get them out for medical treatment. We couldn't use the front door of the compound to get them out because it had bombs in the doorways. When we had gotten in previously, we had to use ladders and climb over the walls. Since the guys were on stretchers in critical condition, we needed to find another way. Will had to blow a hole in the side of the concrete wall with a huge explosive charge.

The enemy seemed to know or expect that we would come out of the hole that was just blown open, and they were ready for us to pop out. I remember there were some local Afghanistan special forces guys who were with us, who had been horrible to work with up to that point. They were lazy and didn't want to do missions or the work. When the chips were down and we were in this situation, they told me through the interpreter, "Hey, whatever happened before, it's done, but we're here together as a team and we're going to fight with you together. Whatever it takes." In their own words they said that they were in this with us, and we could count on them.

When we left the compound, I went with the Afghans first to set security so that the helicopters could land and they could load the patients. The senior guys had given us the game plan for how we were going to set up security. So, we had that plan, and I told the Afghans not to bunch up together, to make sure that they continue to shoot guns in the direction of the enemy, to continue to point toward anything that looked like a fighting position, and not to stop until we got back into the compound. So, we did a 3, 2, 1 countdown and busted out of the hole. It's still one of the craziest experiences that I remember.

The enemy was still waiting for us and as soon as they saw us, they started shooting. They were shooting so much that the field looked like it was on fire. It was fucking insane. So, we set security and started shooting. It blows my mind to remember seeing the

Afghans who we had with us do that day. They performed one heroic act after another. There was so much chaos, and there was so much enemy fire that you would run one step, then have to dive on the ground, zigzag, and do anything you could to be a hard target.

There's No Greater Love Than Somebody Who Will Lay Down His Life for His Friends

Before we even breached the wall, Jack turned to the team and said, "These guys have less than 10 minutes to get on the helicopter in the condition they're in. We're going to have to get them out to the field. Does anyone have a problem risking everything to get them out?"

Not one of us hesitated.

Then he gave us the final instruction, "If you get shot running out to the field, when the helicopter comes, run and get on it."

Two helicopters came down. The first was waved off. The enemy was unloading fire on them, and rocket-propelled grenades (RPGs) screamed through the air. There was no way they could land. But they came back on a second pass. While we waited, we were pinned down by enemy fire in the middle of the field. It was a miracle they made it back and landed. I'm still in awe of the heroic actions that day.

When those of us who stayed made it back to the compound, I remember turning to my buddy and teammate Feez. "What time do you think it is?" we asked each other. We'd been up for days. We guessed 3:00 or 4:00 in the afternoon. It was only 8 a.m.

We were still surrounded. Still fighting to hold the compound. The temperature was already over 100°F and climbing. By midday, it would hit 130°F. It wasn't a good scenario. We ended up fighting all day. We started to run out of water. Eventually, we started running out of ammunition. We'd been dropping bombs all day, burning through round after round, and now we were almost out.

Thankfully, we had outstanding joint terminal attack controllers (JTACs) on our team. They were certified to coordinate with aircraft overhead and call in bomb drops. We were nearly *danger close*, when friendly forces are so close to the target that the risk of friendly fire becomes real. Artillery, air support, naval strikes—everything becomes high stakes.

That's how close they were dropping bombs.

We were still surrounded. Enemy fighters came in packs. All. Day. Long.

The helicopters supporting us overhead were doing gun runs, processing targets that were enveloping us all day long. Large groups of people were running toward us with weapons trying to overrun the compound.

It was probably the hardest, longest day of my entire life. It was a day from hell. Seconds felt like minutes. Minutes felt like hours. It took everything we had just to make it through.

Looking back, this is exactly why we endured hell weeks and all the brutal training. It was to prepare us for moments like this.

> "When surrounded on all sides by seven to eight times our numbers, we faced what seemed the inevitability of death as we attempted the daytime casualty evacuation of our grievously wounded."
>
> —Master Sergeant Brian Jacklin, during his Navy Cross ceremony that included an award ceremony honoring the team's actions

At the end of the night, we were going to be replaced by a Navy SEAL platoon. Jack and Dave, our team's primary JTACs, stayed behind with them. I remember thinking, *How the f*ck are you guys staying out here?*

I hadn't had water in some time and my body was cramped out. My mind and body was f*cked up. My respect to those guys because they stayed there with the SEAL team to support them. The officer of that SEAL team was Dan Crenshaw, now a US congressman from Texas, who lost his eye the next morning from an IED. Somebody in front of him stepped on one and it blew up near Crenshaw and wounded one of his eyes.

Soon after that, we learned our two wounded teammates had been flown to Germany for surgery.

A couple of days later, I spoke with Derek. He had been with us through special ops training in North Carolina. He was the ultimate professional. Always first on the runs, always crushing every standard. He performed at the highest level in everything he did. When I found out he was paralyzed from the chest down, I was devastated.

I could barely form words. All I could get out was, "I don't even know what to say." And Derek, being Derek, said, "Dude, don't worry about it . . . I'm an upper body machine now. I'm going to be good. Just look after the rest of the team and do whatever you need to do to get home."

That was June 14. And we were there until November. So, we still had a long time to survive all the obstacles that would present themselves in the coming months.

This was my third deployment, and I didn't know how many missions I had done, but I had a little experience. To put it into perspective, there are some guys who literally do 20 deployments in special operations. From Marine Raiders, Navy SEALS, Army Special Forces, and Tier 1 guys who do 20+ deployments who are in the mix of these things. There was a young marine on that June 14 mission, and it was his first mission ever. It was his first deployment. Despite the range of experiences, there are many service members who have been overseas and have many events or horror stories under their belts and struggle to integrate, suffer from survivor's guilt, or have other moral or physical injuries that plague them.

Following another training and deployment, I experienced a significant amount of back pain and headaches due to sensitivity to explosions. Even small concussion grenades or gunfire in training environments made my head feel like it would explode. The last school I went to in the military was the Advanced SERE (Survive, Evade, Resist, Escape) school in Spokane, Washington. During the course, I threw my back out. Luckily for me this happened at the end of the course, so the instructors allowed me to stay and graduate. They did make me get an MRI, which revealed a herniated L5-S1 disc in my lower back.

When I returned to my unit, they had gotten the news about my back, and I was sent to medical for extensive tests and assessments.

It was now August 11. We were out on a mission, clearing IEDs, trying to set up a checkpoint for a security position. We had a bunch of marine engineers with us, plus all kinds of gear, and we were trying to take over an old Taliban prison to turn it into a usable site. But the place was full of bombs. We brought in every tool and robot we had to clear them. We even had an excavator scraping explosives off the roof. The bombs just kept going off.

Eventually, the whole building started caving in as the bombs went off. One bomb after another. We couldn't use the building. We spent the entire day trying to secure the area. There were so many explosive devices buried in the ground, rigged in the walls, layered everywhere. The excavator was still working when part of the building collapsed.

As all of this was happening, we heard over the radio that one of the other special operations raider teams that was about 20 miles away was under attack. And we heard that three raiders were killed in an insider attack. At that point, our morale was crushed. We ended our mission for the day and headed back to our compound on our base.

The men killed that day were Gunnery Sgt. Ryan Jeschke, Marine Staff Sgt. Sky Mote, and Capt. Matthew Manoukian. Later, Matthew Manoukian's father was the officiant who married my wife and me. He is a very special person in the Marine Raider community and to all who know him and his family.

It was hard to deal with the fact that three guys were killed in one sitting. The two key leaders on the team both got killed in that event. This was along with the explosive ordnance disposal tech, the bomb technician.

It was a huge loss, but we were still in an environment where we didn't have much time or opportunity to be sad or process these things. We had to keep our guards up high and stay focused. We had to stay alive and keep each other alive. And not just our team but everyone living at our compound. We had army guys, contractors, and interpreters with us. A lot of these people are not fighters, so we had to protect them. You to be ready protect them at a moment's notice when things turned and you were attacked. Sometimes we got attacked every day. At this point we still had several months of survival and fighting left to make it back home.

Insider Attack

On August 13, I was woken up early and told someone was waiting for me outside. I grabbed my interpreter and we went to meet him near the gate compound. It was a guy from the village I'd had some issues with who was always trying to get our attention. I told him to leave and come back in a week, then I went back inside. I sat down at a picnic table, poured some cereal. It was a brutally hot day. August in Afghanistan felt like living in a sauna. I was in board shorts, a muscle shirt, pistol tucked in my shorts, and sunglasses resting on top of my head.

Suddenly, my position exploded. I was blown onto the ground.

I didn't know it at the time, none of us knew it at the time, but one of the Afghan special forces guys had decided to kill everyone inside of our compound. He went up to the tower that they guarded, because he's supposed to protect us from outside, but he decided to actually attack *us* and pointed all the weapons inside on our little compound and started shooting RPGs at me. I was the only one who was outside in the open at that time, so I got hit with the first one. Suddenly I was on the ground and I was delirious.

I remember wondering if a four-wheeler had exploded, or what had happened. I also thought I was blind because my eyes were blacked out. I was holding them open, and I couldn't see. I panicked and wondered if my vision was gone or what the fuck was going on.

Next thing I knew, my vision came back. I was lying there, fully conscious, and I could see again. That's when the chaos really set in. I watched two Afghan special forces guys drop a bag and take off running. Then, there were more explosions, one after another. The whole place was blowing up around me.

After the next explosion, I was able to get into the nearest doorway, the one where my interpreters lived. I had fun relationships with those guys. We had inside jokes and our own weird ways of communicating. When I got inside, they were all huddled together, holding hands and saying, "Big problem . . . big problems."

And yeah, it was serious. But something about the way they said it actually made me laugh a little. That strange humor, that weird little moment, helped me stay calm.

After the initial chaos, I got out and I moved to the operations center, which was right underneath the tower that the Afghan soldier was still shooting out of. Luckily for me, I made it in there without getting hit but I got in there, he started hitting the operation center directly with RPGs. I clearly remember the violence of that sound. Every time one hit, it was an overwhelming, concussion type of feeling where it kind of resets your memory. I clearly remember thinking *What. The. Fuck.* All these explosions were coming in from direct hits, and everything was being destroyed. One of the officers from another unit was under the desk in the fetal position. Two of my teammates were in there, too, and at a certain point an army infantry soldier who was in one of our other security towers came over the radio saying, "Be advised that one of the interpreters is saying that an Afghan special forces guy has gone bad in the tower and needs to be killed."

At this point, now we understood the problem and could work to handle it. Before we thought the enemy had us locked in with mortars, with rockets, or something similar, and were directly hitting us. Our biggest concern was that we didn't know the point of origin of the attacks, which made it scary. Once we knew the attack was coming from the tower, it gave us some confidence to know how to solve the problem.

We cleared our way out of the operations center and got to the back side where all the Afghan special forces guys were. We worked through the problem of getting up to the tower and finishing this guy. He had killed two of his own guys, ones who tried to run up to the tower whom he shot. There were also guys who tried to get up into a position to try to shoot him. He shot them as well. There were three deaths in total.

One thing that still blows my mind is how the shooter let off 12 RPGs in that small of a semi-enclosed space and yet he was still in there shooting his rifle and machine gun at us and at his own guys. By the end of the exchange, the tower was partially on fire and the attacker was killed. Following that, all the other Afghan special forces soldiers who lived with us were traumatized from the event and left our site soon after that.

After the attacks, once we had secured everything, my team took me back to the spot where I was sitting when the attack started. They showed me the RPG. It was right there. There was literally a rocket fin sticking out of the wall directly behind where I had been sitting. Seeing this was significant, and I started to see this event as a miracle. Everything was destroyed around me. There was shrapnel everywhere. My breakfast container with my cereal had shrapnel in it. The table had shrapnel in it right where I was sitting. It was everywhere.

I had been in the kill zone.

I still don't understand how I lived through it.

Afterward, I was in a daze. The days and weeks that followed felt like a blur. Some of my teammates took pictures with me near the picnic table where I'd been blown up. They hugged me, tried to offer comfort, just grateful we survived.

Our medic checked out those of us who got concussions or got fucked up. Some of us got med-evacuated to a larger base. So I was out for a few days, rested up, and then came back to the village, to our team site to finish the rest of the deployment.

Angels in the Battlefield

We had a bunch of other casualties during this deployment. I remember one mass casualty in particular. One of our Afghan checkpoints got hit with a huge explosion. The Taliban drove a motorcycle IED in there, parked it, and waited until everybody was around it. Then they blew it up. More than 30 people were hit and more than 15 people were killed. They brought at least nine patients and all the dead bodies into where we were at. I was there with the interpreter; we were waiting for them to come, and we had a report that the Taliban was trying to hit us with a vehicle IED at the same time.

The interpreter and I had run up to the gate and suddenly there was a vehicle rushing toward us at full speed. It was just the two of us. I had my pistol and my interpreter had an AK-47. The interpreter was a gangster. We yelled for the driver to stop, but the vehicle didn't. The interpreter shot the front of the vehicle with the AK, and the driver finally stopped and put his hands out and said, "Hey, stop! I've got the casualties!"

He brings the bodies up. Most were dead on arrival. Those who were alive we placed in a circle and started working on them. Our other medic Kevin came on the scene. Kevin was a special operations medic like Ginger, an 18 Delta, or 18D.

Both of our medics were amazing. Kevin, aka Big Kev, came in, kept all the patients alive, showed up and did his thing. I just remember working on some of those casualties with him thinking this was what he was born to do. He did an amazing job. He ended up winning the Angels in the Battlefield Award for his work as a special operations medic that year.

In lifeguarding, there's a system that you use when somebody is drowning. You talk to them, saying things such as "You are going to be all right. I'm coming to help you." You call 911, then you go rescue and help that person. I feel like that translates to a lot when you are dealing with casualties in combat, or anyone in a serious medical emergency who requires transportation to a higher echelon of care.

When I sat there with these patients who just had their legs and other parts of their bodies blown off, you know their life is never going to be the same. You are telling them with the interpreter, "Hey, you are going to be all right. You are going to be okay. Help is on the way. The helicopter is coming. You're going to go to a hospital. This is what it's going to be like, you know, you're going to be good. They're going to take care of you."

This particular mass casualty stands out to me. I remember one of the patient's faces and demeanor as I spoke to him to reassure him that he was going to be okay. He looked at me with a blank stare. That look pierced through my consciousness like a subliminal message to me that this war was hopeless and maybe all wars are hopeless.

My main Afghan partner I worked with was our Afghan local police commander, Haji. From the first time I met Haji, I sensed that we would get along well since he had a great sense of humor. He had made the pilgrimage to Mecca, so others look up to him. Along with the influence and power he had in the local area, I quickly understood that culturally it was very important that I had his respect and support in order to effectively lead his local police. With and through Haji, we were able to train and arm nearly 80 Afghan local police. This was the police force that held the security of our small little base, which was essentially reinforced Afghan compounds.

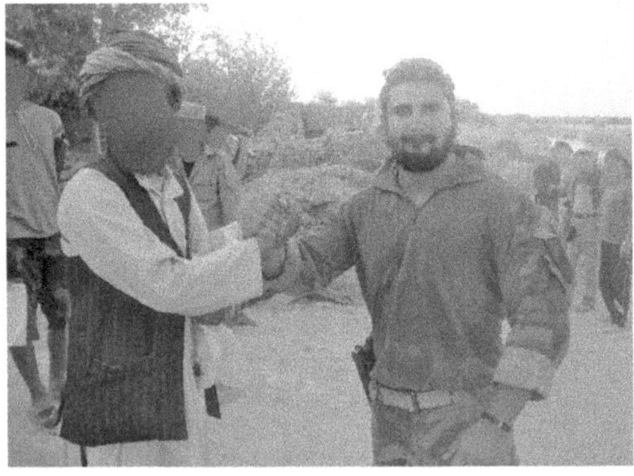

Prime with His Team's Afghan Local Police Commander Haji (2012)

On good days, I remember feeling great when I was able to get my Afghan police more resources such as better weapons, ammo, uniforms, or vehicles. I really cared for a lot of the police force and I also had to keep my head on a swivel the entire time in case any of them turned on me or my team members and clacked off a suicide vest, grenade, or any other course of action that had a potential of happening.

On bad days, there were funerals, mass casualties, deaths. One day toward the end of our deployment in Afghanistan, we conducted training for some of the Afghan police who were preparing to conduct a mission the following day. Haji asked me if he could leave his son with me, which I thought was weird since he had never done that before, but I agreed that he could stay with me until Haji came back later that day.

Haji must have had a sixth sense. When he started his truck and drove away, his vehicle was attacked with a remote controlled IED that had been placed there overnight with an observer who triggered the device to go off. Once Haji's truck drove over the explosives, he was thrown about 20 meters from his vehicle, his legs blown completely off. He still managed to come visit us before we left Afghanistan. He was still in bandages when he visited us.

Toward the end of deployment, we got everything turned over and ready for the next team. We set it up as much as possible to where the next team didn't have to be in that same village. I think they came out to the village for a short period of time, and then they got the transition back to the one of the bases, thankfully.

That was my Afghanistan deployment. I had other deployments, but this was the one that really turned me inside out.

A Warrior's Homecoming (Not Really)

When I returned from Afghanistan, it was funny to me that to get promoted, no matter you just did or whatever you were currently doing, you had to go through a Marine Corps professional education program. This time I had to go to the sergeant's course. I was happy to have a handful of my good Raider buddies with me in this course, including Mike Sims and Jake Cervantes. This was the first time in my whole career that I had female instructors yelling at me and telling me what to do. After being in war, and all that I had been through within the last year, it was extreme culture shock.

Wearing my dress uniform and being evaluated for things like marching and uniform policies, sitting in a classroom felt like we were playing theater arts. I had these instructors; they were in the course, but not necessarily in charge of me. There were times in the first couple weeks when I was missing gear, running late, or something. One of the female instructors liked to yell at me and try to single me out and embarrass me in front of the rest of the group.

Here I was standing in parade rest, which is standing with your hands behind your back, and taking your punishment. And I found this moment to be hilarious because there were a few of us there, coming straight from 360-degree modern warfare, the realest situations where people died every single day. And now were talking about the theory of war, but none of the instructors seemed to have any real-life experience. Not that it matters if you have combat experience, but experience helps if you are teaching classes on warfare, not just teaching something you read in a book.

Instead of getting worked up about this, we decided to have as much fun as we could and make it a vacation. We had a fixed schedule and were getting off at 3 p.m. or 4 p.m. It felt like a break.

The funniest part I remember was on some of the hikes. We climbed these huge hills in Camp Pendleton. We had these progressive hikes, and each week we did more and longer hikes. Anytime I saw a female instructor, I pretended I was too exhausted and I needed to hold onto her pack to make it up the hill. Embracing the absurdity of the situation was my coping mechanism for being in this ridiculous place.

On the final day of the sergeant's course, there is a big celebration called *Mess Night*, where all the marines and instructors wear their dress blues (the fancy uniform) and go to a big formal dinner with a bunch of theatrics. I remember telling the female instructor that night that the reason I had such a hard time in the course was because I was falling for her. She turned completely red and reported me to the senior marine in charge. I was told to report to the sergeant major's office in the morning for my punishment. But we graduated that next day, so I just hid until graduation. My time there came to an end, and I was sent back to my team.

Fast forward. I did another training workup and another deployment. I was at some human intelligence courses, and I had a lot of issues with my back and issues with being around any explosions or training that we were doing in the shoot house, as well the pressure of being around little explosions. Even if it was little concussion grenades that we throw in the house or shooting in training in the house, it made my head feel like it would explode.

I ended up throwing my back out while I was at a school and in a training course in which thankfully I finished, but that was when I got the MRI that showed my L5-S1 disc was blown out.

When I got back from the school and training, I went to medical and a lot of tests and assessments were done on me. I went to an ear, nose, and throat appointment and vestibular appointment where they discovered that I had serious damage in my inner ear. It caused a lot of the pressure and pain that I felt. Ultimately, the combination of traumatic brain injury, my back, and other smaller injuries combined put me on a medical separation board. I was in this separation process for about nine painful months of medical appointments and disability evaluations.

Loss of Identity and Purpose

For me and others on medical separation, it can cause a big identity crisis. One day you go from being a performer and part of something and identifying as a certain way. Then one day you transition out, and suddenly everything is different.

It's the same thing I hear from retiring pro athletes. When they're done fighting in the Ultimate Fighting Championship or playing in the National Football League or their team fires them—whatever the change or end is, but there's something about the day that your jersey gets pulled, or you turn in your gear, and it seems everyone looks at you differently. It's not a comfortable feeling to have your identity stripped, but as they say: as one door closes another door opens. That uncomfortable feeling is energy that can launch you into your next mission.

In hindsight, this was an opportunity to reinvent myself outside of the military. It was a new beginning. It was hard to see at the time, but it was a blessing in disguise. Part of me did not want to leave the military and especially the Raider teams, but it was time for me to start my healing process, even though I had no idea at the time.

Now, I work with a lot of different high-performing individuals, from athletes to CEOs. Through this, I've learned that the life cycle of the role as CEO is about five to seven years. But that's really the life cycle of anyone in any job. Because you might squeeze all the juice out of that one thing for five to seven years and then wonder what's next. And that's how I felt at that time. My life cycle as a Marine Raider lasted eight years, with four years of infantry before that.

I'm grateful that I had the medics and certain people at my unit who looked out for and took care of me. Now there were constant medical appointments for months on end. I was taking all these medications, leading to more appointments, and more medications. It really put me into a low point and dark place.

I was mandated to do a program with the psychologist at the unit, which I didn't feel like I needed. But I was pretty much a robot where I just did everything with a checklist, having little to no emotion about anything. I just did whatever was in front of me on any given day. I was stressed out, but I didn't really have a system to help process what I was feeling and going through.

With the psychologist, I had to do this thing called enhanced exposure therapy—to go through traumatic memories and relive them. I've always been an introverted person, especially then. I was often in flight-or-fight mode when I was in groups or around other people. My psychologist gave me homework assignments to address my social anxiety and trust issues. I was supposed to expose myself in order to reintegrate back into life and not let the things I experienced hold me back. I am grateful for that. But that was just the tip of the iceberg of the work to come as I started to heal.

Prayer

I've never been really complicated with my prayers, but I prayed every day. I've had the same prayer every day since I went to combat, which was always something like this:

> Dear God, thank you for everything. Please forgive me for all my sins. Please help me be a better person. Please keep me and my teammates safe. Amen.

I was praying, but surrender is a powerful thing. And I didn't really know how that worked yet.

Every time I look back and reflect on my life now, I realize I was involved in so many little miracles that leave me wondering how I made it. I know it was not without God and my prayers, and the prayers of all my relatives and prayer warriors back home who were pulling for me to come back safe.

No matter what you are going through, you've just got to know that God has a bigger plan and to surrender to God. In some of my darker days I almost lost my mind to depression, which brought me to the brink of suicide, while trying to figure out the answers to everything that has happened to me, and feeding into negative feedback loops, especially times when I would focus on my survivor's guilt.

I was with some Native Americans recently who had some elaborate prayers and rituals that were so beautiful and they blew me away.

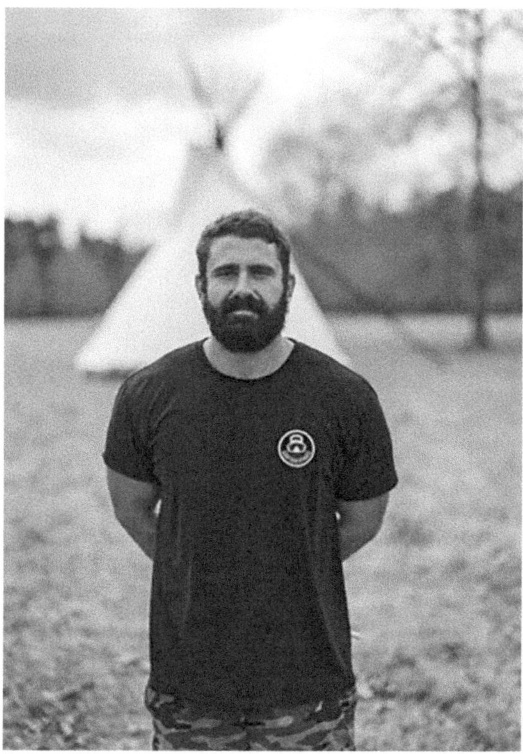

Prime after a prayer ceremony with the Dakota, Chickasaw, and Hopi Native American Tribes

CHAPTER 7

Trusting in Divine Timing

When you open up to healing in your life, it's likely you will experience breakdowns. I believe there are no coincidences in how and when these things happen. It's best to surrender your resistance and make the best choices you can that are based on love, trusting that timing unfolds as part of a divine plan.

I always said I would never get married because I didn't want to end up getting divorced and re-create the wheel that I had experienced. But God and His divine timing intervened and my wife ended up throwing me the life preserver I needed at the time I most needed it.

I was back on the dating scene when I got back from Afghanistan and dated on and off until 2015. I was rarely home in California from 2012–2015, and if I was not deployed overseas, I was usually at some kind of training course and living out of hotels. I was at a point where I was looking for a girlfriend. I had one relationship that created a lot of drama and drag. Then, I was single again and dating, and I was always running into red flags.

I had a couple situations that left me fed up with my experience with dating. At that point I was unable to see the possibility of a relationship for me. I was just over it all and I didn't trust any women. It came down to one week when I had the last drama in a relationship, and I reached a point where I said I was just done dating. I didn't realize it at this time, but this was surrender. It was also divine timing. Because this is exactly when I met my wife, Brittany, in 2015.

Everything happens when it is supposed to happen—not when you want it to happen, and not when you *don't* want it to happen.

Sometimes in life, waiting can feel like you are late or like you missed the timing entirely for meeting goals that you have, or achieving certain milestones in life. It can feel like things are not happening early enough or fast enough. This is something to keep in mind if you find yourself trying to force something and it's just not working out.

The more that I experienced the lows and the highs throughout life, I realized that God makes everything happen when it's supposed to happen. There's a divinity to the ways that make things materialize and manifest. Aligning yourself to God's will for you and your purpose allows for more. This has been my experience. Everyone is on their own journey, but this is something that I feel strongly about.

Instead of forcing something, sometimes it is sitting back and letting things happen. Sometimes things, just like in nature, simply grow. And so however that takes shape in your life with who you are, and what you are doing, things will manifest when you surrender.

In this case, surrender manifested quickly. On December 12, 2015, I was at a paddle party for my good friend Dan Smith. A paddle party is a sacred tradition to send off a Marine Raider getting out of the military. After the party we were at this bar called The Compass, located in Carlsbad, California.

I was not drinking; I was nine years sober at this point. I was just out, playing security and watching over my friends so they did not get in a jam or get in trouble while they were drunk. Some of my friends were talking to a woman and her group of friends, who were partying and having a good time. I could tell this woman was the leader, and she carried a clear confidence; I later learned she owned a salon. I remember I just walked up to her and found out her name was Brittany Adamson. And she went by "Badamson," like she was bad, and I loved it. I grabbed her hand, and she was like, "Woah, what are you doing?!," but she went with it and played along. I got her number that night, and we started to spend time together. Our meeting was really a sign of divine timing and taught me more about surrender.

The timing was important too, because not long after we met, I attended the advanced survive, evade, resist, escape school. I was at an event where I was hurt and threw my back out badly. I had to get MRIs, tests, and scans. The pain was to the point I had trouble walking, sitting, or doing anything that required my back. As I described in Chapter 6, this experience ultimately led me to getting out of the military. The injury and transition came with a lot of challenges and Brittany was really looking out for me while I was going through it.

We moved in together after dating a few months. She had a son, Trey, who had just turned three years old. He was missing a father figure in his life. Trey and I loved having each other around. I consider Trey my son and a godsend. We've grown close over the years, and it's cool because I never thought I would want a relationship with a woman who had a kid, but that was one of the greatest blessings that could have ever happened to me. It was like a two-for-one package deal. While losing my identity as an operator as a result of all the medical challenges, I could lean on them, and they helped give me a new purpose. I felt like Brittany and Trey became my true north. Before meeting her at The Compass, I lacked direction. My compass was constantly spinning, with no meaning to direct me a certain way.

Navigating Transitions

Finding purpose through transition, while also dealing with trauma can be extremely difficult. When you are in an institution like the military, or transitioning from anything where your identity or your purpose comes from being a contributing member of a tribe, or when your purpose and identity are attached to a job that is ending, it needs to be acknowledged in order to transition and find new meaning, purpose, and tribe.

A lot of times, it's not until you transition out that you actually begin to process and face your experiences. This seems especially true for military veterans and first responders. There are a staggering number of suicides. They don't happen while overseas or in the height of battle because you are in survival mode then. They happen later, once back home.

Even if you know that a transition is coming, it can be extremely challenging to redefine what your meaning is and find your new self. Letting go of your old self requires a willingness to let go of attachment.

Realigning might not happen overnight, and a good support system in a time of transition is important. I had a good support system from my unit, like the medical coordinator who made sure all my appointments went right and that people treated me in a somewhat decent way. That really meant a lot. I'm grateful I had people who looked out for me. If they hadn't, I don't know how it would have worked out for me because I was not open to sharing anything with any of my medical doctors; I was in resistance with the world, and I just didn't have the tools at the time to break free of it.

In addition to a support system, seeking education and resources can elevate your life. Sometimes it's formal education, seminars, workshops, or other programs; sometimes it's life school, which is where I know I've learned the most. Life school is continuously putting yourself in more situations to learn and grow. I believe that we all learn more from experiential learning and on-the-job training. If you take the opportunity, you can learn every day from every person you interact with.

When my medical issues came about, I had to think a lot more seriously about what I wanted to do next. These medical issues really crushed my confidence.

My former team leader Derek Herrera had gone through the University of California, Los Angeles master in business administration (MBA) program. I also had other teammates who went to Harvard or other big MBA programs. I decided to start looking at MBA programs as a transition to buy me time to figure out what I wanted to do in life after the military.

One day I got an invite on LinkedIn to go to an info session in Carlsbad for an MBA program. This was perfect because it was just a few miles away from my house. But I had very low self-confidence. I still had a significant workload to finish my bachelor's degree. My benchmark for myself was extremely low. I did not feel worthy of a program like this one. I've shattered that thought process so many times since, but I really had to build myself up to have that confidence to stand in authority of who I am and own what I'm capable of doing.

This invitation came while I was still in the process of being medically separated from the military and several months to go before I finished my bachelor's degree, which was a prerequisite for the MBA program. Between all of this, I was skeptical they would accept my application. I was doubtful they would let me in even if I already had my bachelor's degree.

I was shocked when the administration staff told me I could be accepted for that year if I wanted to commit. I was surprised to receive that opportunity while attending the first info session. I was assured I would be accepted based on my background and leadership experience in the Marine Raiders. I didn't expect that kind of feedback. This was great news. I was really institutionalized, in a comfort zone, and in some ways looking for the next way to fall into another system. I didn't have the confidence of autonomy yet.

Having good mentors and advisors who are looking out for you through any transition period is so important. The same goes for your inner circle and those caring for you while you are going through those transitions and processes.

The timing lined up that when I got out of the military. I would have a couple of months to adjust before starting the MBA program. And right before it started, I had the chance to go to an incredible program called Next Step at Dartmouth. My time there was a breakthrough for me. I was there for three weeks along with other high-level military or Olympians transitioning after their careers. Everyone learned useful skills on how to network and maneuver in a new environment, and how to become more successful, and provided many opportunities. It was very cool to be in that environment and I loved it.

The Call of Entrepreneurship

By the end of the Next Step program there were a lot of opportunities lined up I could have taken, but they were all opportunities to work for other companies. I knew if I tried that path it would not be healthy for me. I knew if I had to fit into a structured box, or work in a cubicle, I would probably flip out all the time trying to deal with fitting in and following rules. I knew I might even end up in jail. Think *Office Space* with potential hostages. At the end of the Next Step course, they had these expert panels. They gathered people from human resources, healthcare, all these different companies or experts from various industries. The group that really spoke to me was the entrepreneurs.

Whenever the entrepreneurs said something, I just felt like I could relate to them, and their stories really lit me up. I had always found ways of earning my own money. I sold candy as a kid, then I went door to door mowing the lawns for anyone I could. My neighbors were my customers. Like most of the entrepreneurs who spoke that day, I'd had a job since I was a little kid. I also resonated with not liking to follow traditional rules. I was actively listening and trying to think seriously about my next steps. And when I heard these guys talk, I knew that I wanted to find something that was going to stretch me and give me purpose the way it did for them. I left the program thinking hard about this.

I was fortunate too that Brittany's parents were very seasoned, successful business consultants. They asked me questions about my passions, skills, and experiences. Where did those things line up with each other? Where did these things intersect? They ran these experience design immersions in Colorado out of their house that were designed for top executives to help them solve strategic problems and reimagine their company from an experience design perspective with the goal for it to be transformative for anyone who interacts with it. I got to go to one of these immersion experiences, and what I worked on throughout that week was figuring out what I was going to do once I transitioned out of the military.

The thing that kept coming up for me was an experiential-based company that changes people's lives. But I wanted it to be something to operate without having any extra fat, removing the risks and costs of any extra overhead or spaces to manage—no brick-and-mortar building. It needed to be successful and make a difference in a big way. I wanted it to be some kind of transformational program and community, an operation that could be run and managed remotely. Centralized planning, decentralized execution just like we did successfully in special military operations. If needed, our headquarters could operate out of a vehicle.

So, I started to put together things I liked to do. I knew I was fascinated by training. I was in all these training sessions—everything from mental focus training, swimming and pool, and coaching. Training others to unlock their potential is something I have been deeply interested in since I started training seriously in 2007. Helping others break through mental and physical barriers aligned with my passion and experience.

Then it became about what kind of training I could offer. I started thinking about how I can take anyone to the gym, and they might have a good time and feel better or more confident, and I can get them to have a breakthrough after a month or couple months of training them. But I knew I wanted something that could change your life in one session. I knew that was going to be something connected with underwater training.

So here I was, about to start my MBA program. My original plan was to build and work with this events company. But I kept thinking back to underwater training and how many breakthroughs we experienced and saw others have in the pool, going outside of their comfort zone to find a new edge. At this time as well, Don Tran was also getting out of the military. We hadn't had much contact since training while in the unit together and we reconnected while we were both getting out. When I talked to Don about these ideas I had, he was immediately aligned. At that time, he wanted to start his own fitness brand. Don has always been an exceptional fitness guy. Sometimes he would max out different things in Raider training, and it would be an outlier number, way above the rest of us. He has always stood out for his fitness and mindset. We started to come up with the plan to launch Underwater Torpedo League and Deep End Fitness, and the rest is history.

The timing was unbelievable. Looking back, all of this feels like part of a plan that was way bigger than us: Don and I went into Marine Raiders at the same time, and now getting out at the same time was a huge gift that allowed us to set up a strong buddy system to handle life outside of the Marine Corps. To have all these things lined up at the same time—to both plan it out and launch it—is crazy to look back at. It reminds me of the saying, "Life is happening for us, not to us."

God's divine timing becomes even more apparent as I look back. Shortly after this time, between transitioning and my reaction to significant amounts of medication, I began to fight some very dark battles internally with depression and mental health.

However a transition takes shape in your life, things will manifest as they are meant to. In life, as you are dealing with transitions, I keep this quote in mind: "The top of one mountain is the bottom of the next. So, keep climbing."

Always build your life for the journey and not the destination.

CHAPTER 8

Hard Drive Reset

When you find yourself at the bottom of your emotional ocean, it may be time for a hard reset. Imagine trying to store five terabytes of data on a one-terabyte drive . . . it's impossible. Similarly, if your mental and emotional mailbox is full, you need to clear space. Recognize when you're overloaded, and take intentional steps to reset, declutter, and focus on what truly matters.

This is especially important in times of major transition, and critical for those transitioning out of the military because that transition is extremely hard. It was very difficult for me after being in for 12–13 years, and I can't imagine how it goes for somebody after being in for 20 years or longer with copious amounts of trauma from war, plus their childhood on top of that.

When you are part of an institution like the military, you surrender your autonomy, so regaining a sense of control over your life takes serious effort. It is important to redirect and reposition yourself for the future that you want. It's a challenge to begin figuring out who you are and take risks to find yourself. To evolve, it's necessary to let go of whatever attachment you have from who you were before in the military (or whatever it is you are leaving behind). There were a lot of times that I felt lost, letting that former part of myself go. Now I realize that was necessary to reach new potential in my life.

While in the military, it's easy to get institutionalized. I am not talking about brainwashing here. That's something completely different. We see this when service members get out, like a prisoner who adapts so much to being inside a cell that they don't know what to do when they are out. It's hard to live, work, and operate outside of that regimented system. It's basically a military version of *The Shawshank Redemption.* In the military, you get paid every two weeks by the government, sometimes for 20+ years. It can be scary to leave that. I see so many people struggle to find their true self when they get out, just like I did.

Your comfort zone and reputation are built behind the positions you've had. It can become a huge attachment. I'm not saying any of that is right or wrong. From a growth perspective, it's hard to grow when you stay in the same place or environment.

I had my own comfort zone that was built behind the varied positions and experiences I had in the military. This created a huge attachment for me. For a short period of time, I even tried to stay in. I thought my biggest opportunity would be to reenlist, get a reenlistment bonus, and stay in for another four years. I didn't have a clue then that everything my life holds today would even be possible. Had I known, it would have been smoother sailing for me.

If your military duty included trauma, it can be difficult to process it, taking what is already a critical time for many to a greater level of challenge. For those leaving the military or special operations, you may be contending with operator syndrome. According to the National Library of Medicine, operator syndrome is understood to be the natural consequences of an extraordinarily high allostatic load; the accumulation of physiological, neural, and neuroendocrine responses resulting from the prolonged chronic stress; and physical demands of a career with the military special forces. Clinical research and comprehensive, intensive immersion programs are needed to meet the unique needs of the members of this community.

Rapid Response Therapy

For me, when I got out of the military, I was really closed off. I felt like a robot who didn't have access to my emotions. I lived in a checklist mentality. I just did thing after thing, every day, without processing or thinking much. I entered a new phase with my family. I was newly married, a father to Trey, and Brittany was pregnant; we had a baby girl on the way. There was so much change, and at the same time I hadn't processed any of my trauma from the military or childhood yet. I was also going through a period of rediscovering myself. The things I liked or assimilated with in the military weren't things that I liked when I got out. This was not smooth for me.

It was a lot to deal with and adjust to in general, not to mention all the medical appointments and side effects from all the medications I was on. The list was growing. Despite moving my life forward from the military in so many ways, I was suffering mentally and emotionally.

About this time, I saw that one of my teammates from my team in Afghanistan was really struggling. He had a lot of trouble in life, was living on the streets, and had gotten a bull's-eye tattooed on his forehead. He had me really worried. I found a nonprofit that offered a treatment called rapid response therapy (RRT) that I thought could help him. I showed it to him, and he responded positively to it. We got him signed up and purchased plane tickets to Florida, where the program was located. We were both supposed to go so I could support him.

He never showed up, and I ended up there by myself. I told them I didn't know why he wasn't there. As I was preparing to leave, they said, "No you're going to do the treatment instead."

"Nah, I don't need to do this," I responded. I was resistant and not open—I had a fixed mindset—to the idea of doing this myself. They pressed further saying, "Why don't you just try it since we have all of the support and therapists already here," and they convinced me to try. So that week, I ended up doing this RRT, which set me on a healing path and altered my life forever.

RRT uses guided imagery, hypnosis, storytelling, and other forms of talk therapy to resolve troubling thoughts, feelings, and behaviors related to your trauma. RRT was developed to treat combat veterans and sexual abuse victims. RRT continues to spread as a healing modality to other communities and populations to heal trauma.

Essentially, you are hypnotized, and then the therapists go in and start finding the memories and the data files inside your conscious or subconscious that are bothering you, and then they start to try and clean that up.

For me, the first day was spent revisiting all military-related memories. I felt a huge shift right away. I felt more present. I remember looking out the windows and noticing the grass, plants, and all of nature so much more clearly and just being in awe of the world around me. I saw things differently. Somehow, I could see more colors.

I built a good rapport with my therapist, Dr. Mike Cortina from Chicago, and gained a lot of respect for him. There was a lot of trust there. And on the second day, I came in and he said, "Prime, man, you got so much done yesterday. You were so focused. Once we got to work, you worked through things like boom, boom, boom. What do you want to work on today?"

To that point, I hadn't really talked about my childhood or done anything about it, ever. I don't know what triggered me to open that can of worms. But I said, "I think I want to look into my childhood."

They put me under hypnosis again on the second day, and we started to deal with experiences from when I was a child. We began to dive into all the scarcity, abuse, peeping Tom, and deep-seated trauma that I stuffed down into my subconscious. It was buried very deep. This was a gift and a curse to unlock these memories. It was good because this started me on my healing journey, but now conscious awareness of my experiences began to drive me crazy at the same time.

Pandora's Box

RRT opened a lot for me, in a positive direction and in a healing way. But also it opened what I call my Pandora's box: the things that I had buried. These memories now felt fresh on the surface. Fresh and raw.

I was and still am a super introverted person. I didn't like being in a room full of people. As I left Florida to return to California, I felt people's energy around me, which was new and overwhelming. I remember the colors were shockingly vivid at the airport and when looking out the windows from the plane. Before this treatment, I experienced things as dark, bland, and dull. I wore nothing but black. And after, all the colors were vivid and alive to me. These changes were lasting. Now, I'm a little more into wearing and embracing the full spectrum of color. This experience speaks to the brain's neuroplasticity when processes are followed to enhance it. It was different and overwhelming, and I was not always stable, sometimes breaking down entirely.

I was about to begin the master of business administration (MBA) program and being in groups of people was a part of it. Everything was compounding. It felt like my hard drive was full and walls were closing in on me. I thought the only way I could get through the MBA program was if I allowed myself to drink through it. I made up my mind that I couldn't do it sober.

I had been sober for 10 years while I was in the marines. I do not think I would have made it into special operations if I had not gotten sober the first time. I never would have unlocked my potential because I know that drinking is toxic for me. I have a lot of alcoholism in my family, but now I have awareness that when I drink, it's like Dr. Jekyll and Mr. Hyde, and my shadow self comes out and I get in trouble. It just drags me down.

So here I was, out of the military, in my MBA program, I was just starting Deep End Fitness (DEF) and Underwater Torpedo League (UTL) with Don. The pressure of these different stressors built up and I was drinking again.

I started to have these thoughts about my childhood and replaying parts of it in my head. I also replayed things I had seen in war. It was all looping repeatedly. More of these thoughts were coming to my head and I was having a really hard time controlling them.

With these thoughts, the stressors of life, my MBA program, and the businesses, plus all the medical, psych, and Post-Traumatic Stress appointments with the Veterans Administration (VA), my mental health really suffered. It started to affect me in a catastrophic way. In hindsight, I can see that I was not doing the work to integrate these traumas, or the maintenance to take care of myself and my mental health. I was lost and didn't have the tools yet to cope and navigate the emotions I was experiencing.

At first, I just wasn't willing to play a victim role. So, I shut it down as much as I could, saying, "Nah, I'm not a victim. I am not playing these victim games." Over time, slowly but surely, the victim story started coming into my mind, with two main themes that triggered these thoughts. One of the themes concerned my traumas from childhood, and the other was survivor's guilt and questioning the meaning of the wars, especially Afghanistan.

I ended up in a loop of "why me?" If you are not careful and you start asking "why me" or "why us" or "why that" it becomes a trap that is easy to get caught into.

This is when I started experiencing the "why me?" feedback loop. The things that were coming up for me from my childhood and other trauma and I identified how it was holding me back.

Maybe I needed to go through this experience of overcoming the victim loop to get to where I am now. I should have looked at some of these traumas I faced earlier in life. But I appreciate what I've learned from going through the experience of identifying the feedback loops and learning how to deal with them and break through to the other side.

I came to realize that these events empowered me for my future. I also know how to relate to others who are facing this because I have been in that mindset myself.

Moral Injury

Derek Herrera told me several years ago something that has supported my survivor's guilt. "Dude, do you think any of the guys we lost in Afghanistan would feel any better if you were any more messed up than you are now?" This has been one of the most powerful reframes I have experienced.

DEF and UTL

It's interesting because as I was moving into my post-military purpose, I started having breakdowns at the same time.

My mother-in-law, Leezy, aka Bonus Mom, kept telling me, "Your purpose is where your passions intersect with your experience and interests, and how that can translate into a paying profession."

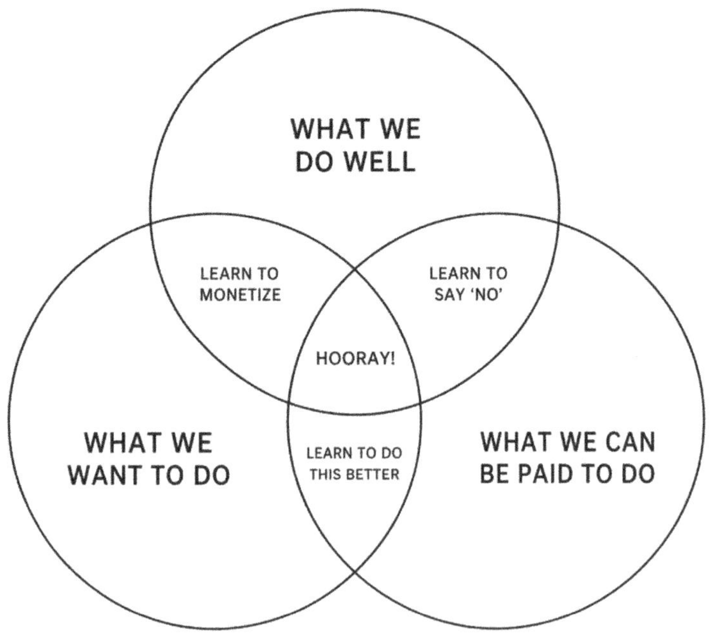

Every time I thought about my answer to this, I thought about how much I loved to see people reach their breakthroughs. I like helping people unlock potential, and how water confidence and performance training was something I could do to help someone achieve a huge transformation in one day or even one hour.

In some ways I had been forming this idea in my head for UTL for a long time—years at this point.

I first became fascinated and intrigued with something we played called underwater football back when I worked at the pool on base. It quickly became my favorite thing to do. I loved to take the torpedo, which we used as the football, and get as many people as possible to try and tackle me underwater.

It quickly became my favorite thing to do. At end of my Iraq deployment when I trained at an indoor swimming pool at the Al Asad Airbase, I remember photos on the wall of Navy SEALS and marine recon teams competing against each other in water polo. These photos got me thinking, *why aren't they playing underwater football?*

It was a super creative and empowering activity, and I've since seen how this sport and this game can unlock results for people. The goal was always to break away from everybody and make the score. One of my favorite parts of UTL is that if a defender grabs you underwater while you have the torpedo, you can start a spin move. They almost have to let go of you, which gives you the ability to break free and make a play.

In the marines, we worked our asses off. All week long, all day, each day. Sometimes 16–20 hours a day. Often, we had to work on the weekends pulling guard or standing duty. Other times we got the full weekend off. It just depended on what was going on.

The main thing I did to recover was go to the pool in town. I'd float in and go under the water and think and just be there by myself. I kept imagining teams playing this game as a sport.

So when I started the MBA program, it was something in the background of my mind for about 10 years before I got out of the military. And every time I got a chance to speak to my class and professors about UTL and DEF, I did. I researched the landscape of underwater sports and found that this is an Olympic-like sport in nature. A gladiator sport that didn't exist yet.

Don and I started UTL with two pools. We had one pool in Oceanside, in North San Diego, and one in San Clemente in Orange County. We set up the pools for two months each to run as a test period to see if we could get two full teams to train and participate in the Aqua Bowl Championship, our Superbowl for UTL.

We originally named it the Underwater Football League. In doing research, I found there was an Underwater Football League in Canada. But it was different from ours. They play with a neutrally buoyant ball and they use fins. Our version requires no fins and requires all natural swimming abilities; additionally, we use a torpedo, which can glide across half the length of a pool in one pass. We also use the entire pool, from all angles. It's a 360° sport because attackers can come from any angle, and the plays are not just at the bottom of the pool. It makes for a very dynamic, fast-paced, and innovative sport.

When we launched the Underwater Football League, within a few weeks we had gotten so many hits about "where's the football" or "why is it called football, you don't use a football," so within weeks we changed to UTL, and we have been running with it ever since.

As an introvert, I've never really felt like a big presenter or a natural at being in front of people, or so I thought. As we launched the companies, it was an obstacle and opportunity for me to get outside of my comfort zone. An opportunity to get a lot reps with presenting because that's what you have to do when launching something like this.

While all of this was going on, I was working with my mentor, Derek Herrera, who had been shot in Afghanistan and was paralyzed from the chest down. He was now running his first medical device company and mentoring me as I transitioned out of the military and I was getting into my MBA. We decided to start a nonprofit event, called the Marine Raider Challenge.

The Marine Raider Challenge was an off-base event that special ops guys could participate in to honor their fallen teammates and to bring together families and relatives of fallen service members. I was the director of this nonprofit, and I consistently ran the event

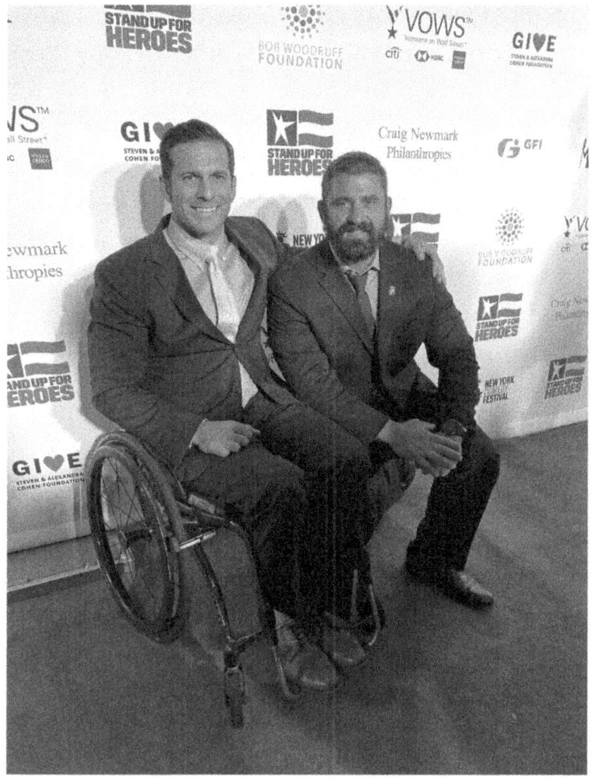

Prime with His Mentor Derek Herrera

annually as well as other events, which required me to go to a lot of city planning meetings in San Clemente (not my favorite activity or how I wanted to spend my time). I also had to deal with officials who tried to shut down our event due to politics and procedure, and I had to work to keep it on.

Feedback Loops

There was a lot that kept me busy, but in the background, I was having more breakdowns. My negative thoughts and feedback loops were challenging to deal with, and transition became much more difficult than I ever imagined it could be. At a certain point, I began to identify two feedback loops that were driving me crazy.

First, why did I have the childhood that I had growing up? My son was now seven years old at this time. Seeing him around the same age that I was when I experienced some of my most traumatic events triggered me. I'd think, *How did this happen to me? Nothing like this would ever happen for my kids. If something like this happened to my son, it would be game over. How did it happen to me for years? How did somebody watch me from a window and I hid for so many years in my closet?*

The second loop was *Why and how did I survive the enemy attacks, and why am I still here? Why did I get hit with rocket-propelled grenades and I am still here but not others?*

I didn't realize that these were victim mindsets. I was stuck in my feedback loops. I replayed these events over and over again in my mind and I created superhighways in my mind with these stories. I was obsessed with thinking about them. They were on repeat in my mind. Then I would drink and it would feel even more compounded. Eventually, I started to experience my mental health crashing. I was aware that something was seriously off or "not normal" for how I was feeling. I clearly knew something was wrong when I found myself prescribed between 15 and 20 medications for depression, headaches, and so on. At the time it seemed normal since I saw and heard about so many of my friends transitioning out and being put on a slew of different meds to manage pain, anxiety, headaches, and post-traumatic stress.

I was on so many pills. This is just one page of 13 pages of what I was prescribed throughout this time.

About this time, I made the decision to go off all my pharmaceutical meds and transitioned to plant-based medicine, which worked for me at the time. But I was also drinking again, and after 10 years of being sober, I went completely off the rails and drank excessively. This was not a great combination. I wouldn't suggest anyone to take pharmaceuticals to begin with if you can help it because when you stop, you feel everything.

When I got off anti-depressants, I experienced everything and feel all the emotions that were previously blocked by the meds. Today, I don't want to mask or block it out. But at the time I wanted to mask it.

TRAMADOL (ULTRAM) 50MG ORAL TABLET--PO 5 TAKE 1 TO 2 TABLETS BY MOUTH EVERY SIX HOURS AS NEEDED FOR PAIN #40 RF0
Taking: No Origin: DoD Refills Left: NR; Last Filled on Not Recorded; Ordered By: HUGHES,STEPHEN MCBURNEY ; Order Start Date: 07 Oct 2016; Order Expires on 12 Oct 2016; NMC San Diego; Order Number: 161007-08137;
Status: (Out) Discontinued

ZOLPIDEM TARTRATE (AMBIEN) 10MG ORAL TAB TAKE ONE TABLET BY MOUTH EVERY NIGHT AS NEEDED FOR SLEEP #10 RF0
Taking: No Origin: DoD Refills Left: NR; Last Filled on Not Recorded; Ordered By: LIU,JIE , Order Start Date: 30 Sep 2016; Order Expires on 30 Oct 2016; NMC San Diego; Order Number: 160930-09847;
Status: (Out) Discontinued

MELOXICAM (MOBIC) 15 MG ORAL TABLET--PO TAKE ONE TABLET BY MOUTH EVERY DAY WITH FOOD AS NEEDED FOR PAIN #90 RF0
Taking: No Origin: DoD Refills Left: NR; Last Filled on Not Recorded; Ordered By: VILLARROEL,MICHAEL LOUIS ; Order Start Date: 02 Sep 2016; Order Expires on 01 Dec 2016; NMC San Diego; Order Number: 160902-10973;
Status: (Out) Discontinued

RIZATRIPTAN (MAXALT) 10MG ORAL TABLET TAKE ONE TABLET BY MOUTH AT START OF HEADACHE , MAY REPEAT IF NO EFFECT AFTER 2 HOUR MAX 2/DAY OR 10/WEEK #1 RF0
Taking: No Origin: DoD Refills Left: NR; Last Filled on Not Recorded; Ordered By: LIU,JIE ; Order Start Date: 24 Aug 2016; Order Expires on 08 Oct 2016; NMC San Diego; Order Number: 160824-20006;
Status: (Out) Discontinued

TOPIRAMATE (TOPAMAX) 25MG TAB TAKE TWO TABLETS BY MOUTH TWICE A DAY #120 RF2
Taking: No Origin: DoD Refills Left: 2 of 2; Last Filled on Not Recorded; Ordered By: CHUNG,JAMES ; Order Start Date: 12 Aug 2016; Order Expires on 12 Aug 2017; NMC San Diego; Order Number: 160812-14121;
Status: (Out) Discontinued

RIZATRIPTAN (MAXALT) 10MG ORAL TABLET TAKE ONE TABLET BY MOUTH AT START OF HEADACHE , MAY REPEAT IF NO EFFECT AFTER 2 HOUR MAX 2/DAY OR 10/WEEK #1 RF0
Taking: No Origin: DoD Refills Left: NR; Last Filled on Not Recorded; Ordered By: KELLER,MATTHEW WILLIAM ; Order Start Date: 10 Aug 2016; Order Expires on 24 Sep 2016; NMC San Diego; Order Number: 160810-08474;
Status: (Out) Discontinued

TRAMADOL (ULTRAM) 50MG ORAL TABLET--PO 5 TAKE 1 TO 2 TABLETS BY MOUTH EVERY SIX HOURS AS NEEDED FOR PAIN #60 RF0
Taking: No Origin: DoD Refills Left: NR; Last Filled on Not Recorded; Ordered By: HUGHES,STEPHEN MCBURNEY ; Order Start Date: 27 Jul 2016; Order Expires on 26 Aug 2016; NMC San Diego; Order Number: 160727-16182;
Status: (Out) Discontinued

METHYLPREDNISOLONE DOSEPAK 4MG TAB--PO 4 TAKE AS DIRECTED IN PACKAGE #21 RF0
Taking: No Origin: DoD Refills Left: NR; Last Filled on Not Recorded; Ordered By: HICKEY,ANITA H , Order Start Date: 18 Jul 2016; Order Expires on 17 Aug 2016; NMC San Diego; Order Number: 160718-15874;
Status: (Out) Discontinued

TRAMADOL (ULTRAM) 50MG ORAL TABLET--PO 5 TAKE 1 TO 2 TABLETS BY MOUTH EVERY SIX HOURS AS NEEDED FOR PAIN #60 RF0
Taking: No Origin: DoD Refills Left: NR; Last Filled on Not Recorded; Ordered By: VILLARROEL,MICHAEL LOUIS ; Order Start Date: 15 Jul 2016; Order Expires on 23 Jul 2016; NMC San Diego; Order Number: 160715-09273;
Status: (Out) Discontinued

TOPIRAMATE (TOPAMAX) 25MG TAB TAKE ONE TABLET BY MOUTH EVERY NIGHT FOR SEVEN DAYS AND INCREASE BY ONE TABLET AS TOLERATED EVERY WEEK TO A MAXIMUM OF FOUR TABLETS BY MOUTH EVERY NIGHT FOR NEUROPATHIC PAIN, DECREASE FREQUENCY AND INTENSITY OF HEADACHES. #120 RF0
Taking: No Origin: DoD Refills Left: NR; Last Filled on Not Recorded; Ordered By: VILLARROEL,MICHAEL LOUIS ; Order Start Date: 08 Jul 2016; Order Expires on 07 Aug 2016; NMC San Diego; Order Number: 160708-06907;
Status: (Out) Discontinued

LIDODERM 5% PATCH (LIDOCAINE) APPLY ONE PATCH EVERY DAY AS NEEDED 12 HOURS ON 12 HOURS OFF #30 RF0
Taking: No Origin: DoD Refills Left: NR; Last Filled on Not Recorded; Ordered By: HUGHES,STEPHEN MCBURNEY ; Order Start Date: 17 Jun 2016; Order Expires on 17 Jul 2016; NMC San Diego; Order Number: 160617-10054;
Status: (Out) Discontinued

TRAMADOL (ULTRAM) 50MG ORAL TABLET--PO 5 TAKE 1 TO 2 TABLETS BY MOUTH EVERY SIX HOURS AS NEEDED FOR PAIN #30 RF0
Taking: No Origin: DoD Refills Left: NR; Last Filled on Not Recorded; Ordered By: HUGHES,STEPHEN MCBURNEY ; Order Start Date: 17 Jun 2016; Order Expires on 21 Jun 2016; NMC San Diego; Order Number: 160617-10021;

Launching DEF

During summer 2018 we were running DEF and UTL, and momentum really started building. We got hit up by an offseason NFL trainer, Richard Power, to run a six-week course. At first, I trained people who contacted us on social media or online, and the first year we were experimenting/beta testing, so with Rich this was the first big push with training elite athletes. We created a huge buzz over this six-week course.

After this, Coach Marsh, one of the best swim coaches of all time, heard about what we were doing with the program and observed us training. Then we started working with him. He brought a lot of athletes who are getting ready for the 2020 Olympic games.

We worked with Manti Te'o, an NFL player. Ilima Lei MacFarland, the MMA Bellator flyweight champion, had a fight camp, and she started bringing out these different Ultimate Fighting Championship fighters, like Liz Carmouche, who were in San Diego. Our work really challenged the athletes and took them to new levels with their mental focus, breathing, and recovery. This momentum continued to build, and we were now working with an array of professional athletes and Olympians. We also worked with challenged athletes as well as individuals who had had a stroke or maybe lost limbs overseas. I had found a lot of purpose in all the work we were doing.

I became more obsessed with human performance. What works, what doesn't? How can I unlock more results? I trained different athletes and helped them reach breakthroughs that helped in their highest moments of performance.

After the training sessions, I would go to my car and notice tears rolling down my face. This kept happening more frequently. I was in a deep and dark depression, but I was hiding it. My wife could tell, and so could Nana, my grandmother. I kept it hidden otherwise and people didn't know. One of the sayings in the marines that was engrained in me was "suffer in silence," and this is pretty much what I was doing. I had become an expert at this, but it was killing me from the inside out.

I also attended a six-month incubator/business accelerator program. This *Shark Tank*–like program coincided with my MBA program, while running the nonprofit and starting the businesses. In this program they assigned each of us seven business professional advisors who worked with me for a year and helped us get DEF ready to scale. This felt like a full-time job itself. I was doing so much real-life stuff that school seemed to be my last priority. It was just another thing to take care of on top of all these other things I was responsible for. And to go do something like an academic assignment was not on my priority list because I had real-life challenges to work through and take care of, as well as fighting the underlying serious problem of my mental health.

Between these breakdowns and everything I was balancing, I had to weigh what was most important to prioritize. It would have a more negative impact if I didn't meet the requirements for the incubator, the nonprofit, and my work, than it would be for getting a lower grade on an assignment. When we started the MBA program the staff had informed us that the importance of the program was to build a strong network and that grades were not as important as having a powerful community of like-minded leaders to tap into long after the program ends.

It was chaotic at that time, I felt like there was an overload of mental tabs open.

How it would materialize would be struggling with quizzes and assignments, and missing deadlines or things that other people in the program were working on all week. I had to knock things out in the lobby right before classes, trying to get things done in 5–10 minutes, surrendering to whatever grade I got. Eventually I landed on academic probation.

Looking back, I was not a good teammate and was probably more of a distraction with my behavior and mental state than a value add. I was the cause and source of all the problems I had at the time. It's not that the program was bad. It was a great program and not overwhelmingly difficult. It was just the situation that I had created.

I take responsibility. I was the one who created the circumstances, and I was responsible for getting myself out of it, but I had no idea how or what to do to make positive changes. I was about to do my final project, but unfortunately, I had a breakdown and a fallout with my team. There were conflicts with others in the MBA program who really cared about the grades and put tons of time into it. I didn't care as much, or at all, because I was in fight or flight. Grades were one of my last priorities.

I left my MBA team before we presented the final project. I was in a predicament because I was on academic probation and this assignment was a big part of the grade, so it was a big deal. I contemplated dropping out of school. There were seven other former marines in the program, too. They all individually reached out and asked how they could support. "We're not letting you do this on your own. Whatever you need, we're going to make sure you're good and able to graduate." And it was cool to receive that support.

The other thing that was neat was that the faculty and staff all voted every year for the top MBA student, who then goes up for the top 100 MBA in the country, called Poets & Quants. I have no idea why, but the staff had voted for me. I got a call from one of the administration members who called me to say (1) I was off academic probation and (2) I was nominated by my professors and the academic staff for being one of the top 100 MBAs in the country.

I was confused because of my grades and asked them how this was possible. They said it about what I was doing and building in life. Not to worry about the grades, because what I was building was what it's all about. This is what encouraged me to ride out the last couple of months of the program. Many of the students had my back as well as the faculty and administrators.

Too Many Open Tabs

The obstacle for me was that I was at the end of my MBA program, and there were a million things going on. When there were so many tabs open, it was hard to be present or have a deep level of focus on *any*thing. Before I dove into the healing work and opened the Pandora's box of my traumas, I was just living on the surface. Yes, I was living life, watching sports, and so on, but I did not fully experiencing the highs and lows. I kept the eruption of memories that were replaying in my mind to myself as much as possible and stayed right there on the surface. Until they could not be stuffed away anymore.

The breakdowns, drag, and feedback loops basically created an awakening and unlocked crazy opportunities for me to have a deeper connection and meaning in life. It's opened the way for deeper relationships, conversations, and trust. Trust has always been a big thing for me, ever since childhood and then being in the inside attack, where the people I trusted (to a certain extent) tried to *kill* me. It's hard for me to trust anyone. Over time, I've developed an openness to taking risks and I've made gains as a human, and connection and relationships with others, which has led me to discover even more of my true purpose and meaning in life. These things gave me the encouragement to open up and tell my story, which led to writing this book.

I knew I needed to do something. I was in a serious breakdown. I didn't like going to the VA. From my perspective it always seemed more about the disability benefits, not about actually helping you get better or with your healing. Instead, it felt like a trap. After a lengthy process I got accepted into Operation Mend, which is a charity for special operations veterans who are not getting the support they need from the VA. It's an amazing program with a lot of high-level support from University of California, Los Angeles (UCLA) and the UCLA medical team. I went there for a lot of assessments ahead of a six-week in-patient mental health program.

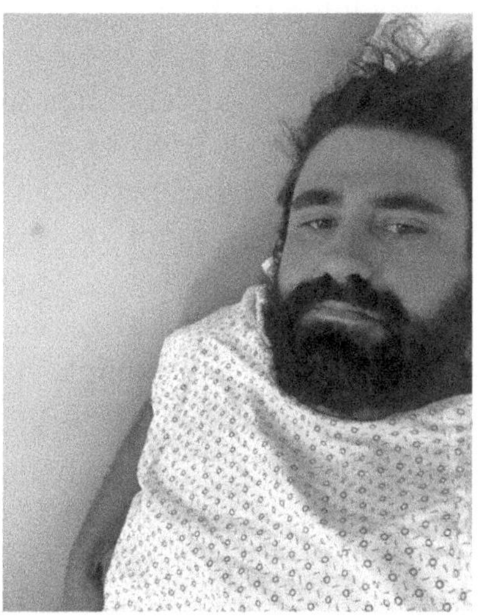

Prime at UCLA medical center
undergoing medical tests (2018)

When I went to my appointments for Operation Mend, I would stay in a hotel and then find the worst areas and neighborhoods of Los Angeles (LA) and just walk around all night long. Looking back, it's hard to explain why I did that, but I just wanted to be put in the realest of situations I could find. I felt like a lot of life was artificial, and at that time, suburban life did not add up to me or make sense to me. I felt like I was losing my mind.

Toad Journey

Brittany had been super concerned about me for a while. And it got to this point where I had the six-week Operation Mend in-patient program coming up, but it wasn't going to start for a month still.

There were some healers through these special operations networks that had been reaching out to me for months trying to get me into a healing journey. I had been hearing stuff on podcasts about Mike Tyson doing 5-MeO-DMT and how it had transformed and changed his life in just one session and treatment.

Even though I was interested because of what I heard about Mike Tyson, I kept blowing it off. It seemed like it was going to be this networking thing because they kept saying that this or that famous person would be there. I was in full breakdown and not interested in anything like that; I was not interested in any games or anything fake.

One day my buddy Myles, who had been sending me all this information, asked me why I said no to everything. What was going on?

"I have serious problems, I don't need to go to any networking thing. I don't want to do this with other people. If I am going to do something like this, I need to do it isolated, by myself."

Myles asked if I would be open to trying to go to a private one in LA the following weekend. It would just be me and a couple of civilians. I agreed that felt like a better setting to me.

It's strange. I was in such a breakdown in my life. And at that time, for some reason I had packed a bag and kept it in my car. I felt like I was going to jail. Or going away somewhere I didn't know. It's hard to explain where my head was at.

I was in such deep depression, with tears coming uncontrollably at all times, and not knowing what to do. I just tried to keep myself busy with work and school, so I had to take some precautions because I was not stable. I had to get rid of my gun that was in my house. I had to create these anchors for myself. My daughter was one year old at this time, and I kept her teddy bear in my car to anchor myself, to remind myself not to do something traumatic. I even went to lunch every week with my mother-in-law, Leigh. Those lunches were another big anchor point. I had a lot of raw conversations; I was at the end of my rope with everything, and I could not hide it anymore.

I felt like I was in the passenger seat of my own life, not the driver's seat. I was detached. I was not in control. And that was when it started to feel really scary. The healing journey with Operation Mend was set up, but it was still weeks away. On one particularly bad day, Brittany came home and asked me, "What are you going to do?"

I told her I had something lined up in two weeks. "I don't think you can make it through this weekend. You need to do something *now.*

I don't think you can wait two weeks with how you are operating right now. You need to figure it out and call them and see what you can do *this weekend*." I realize now that what I was going through was extremely challenging on her as well.

I called the healer and explained where I was at, and asked, "Whatever you have on the West Coast, can I come this weekend? I'll fly there or drive there. Whatever you have. I need help now."

He responded positively, "Yes, we're going to be in Northern California on Saturday. Be there by 11 a.m. Here's what to bring," and he proceeded to give me a starter kit of things to read ahead of time and what to know.

At that time, I didn't have much, if any spiritual awareness. I was all ego, and I was in breakdown. I was losing my mind, but I already had a bag packed.

The next day, I said goodbye to my family and drove up to Northern California. As I drove, everything within me was at a boiling point. I kept reliving being in explosions and being in an insider attack.

I thought about how being around loud noises would ruin my day and put me into fight or flight and acknowledged that I was in full depression. That being around people was draining. I couldn't stop these memories from childhood playing in loops in my head.

Setting Intentions

As I drove to the location, feeling all these different emotions, it was overwhelming.

At one point, I pulled over on the side of the road, got out of my car, and took off on a sprint. I hadn't run in two years, I had an injury on my foot, but here I was running, screaming, and yelling, "I can't do this shit anymore. I am done!" I kept repeating, "I am done!"

I didn't know anything about setting intentions yet, which is such a big part of working with plant medicine and healing journeys. You set an intention and that carries you into the journey. Intentions are the energy of the soul. I knew a lot of what was bothering me, but I didn't know how to let go of any of it.

I wasn't aware at the time, but I did set an intention of surrender. I just knew I needed to reset. I wanted to heal and move forward and let go of all this shit that I didn't even know was bothering me, things I didn't have the tools to process or deal with. I was at a full surrender point in life, waving the white flag and feeling like I didn't have the tools to break through. I was so vulnerable that I was open to doing this powerful healing experience as I had no other options. This was it.

That night, I stayed at a hotel and the next morning, I drove the last couple of hours. I remember I was scared about what was going to happen when I got there. But knowing that Mike Tyson did it, and had these transformational experiences, I knew it was going to help me. I had a lot of fears and anxiety about it, but I kept going.

As I got close to the house, I had a lot of fight or flight and resistance; I was looking for excuses to leave. But there were little signs that kept me moving forward. Just before I made my final turn to go toward the house, a little girl in the backseat of the car ahead of me waved at me through the window, and she reminded me of my daughter. She smiled like it was going to be okay. And it just gave me this peace and assurance that I was going to the right place, a sign that I needed to keep going.

I pulled up to the gate, which was beautiful. It looked like something out of a kid's book. I was just struck by its beauty. I put in the gate code and it opened just like magic. And Master Adeon, a small man, maybe 110 lbs., dressed in full robes came out. He looked and sounded like an Australian Jesus.

He's said, "Hey, brother, you made it. Everything is okay. We're all in the back. So, whenever you are ready, you can just come back."

Then he asked me, "Are you going to stay here with us tonight?" I was at the end of myself, not able to look past the present moment, and said, "I don't know anything that I am doing. I am just doing this one thing at a time. I don't know where I am staying tonight. I don't care." I had no plan for after this.

He gently said, "It's okay, it's okay. No worries."

There were some apprentices there helping with the ceremony, which was being held for me and one other person. I followed one of them to the back and we're on this magical piece of land. There was a beautiful rose garden to the right and a swimming hole in front of us. There were little chairs shaped and painted like mushrooms around where were going to do the healing circle.

It looked like a setting from a fantasy fairy tale. The healers were dressed in robes, and it looked like a mystical place. I had never seen anything like this before, and it was so far out of context for my life, it was already blowing my mind just being there.

When the ceremony began, they blessed us and cleansed the space. They opened the container for healing. Then, we got further into the ceremony, and they gave us instructions for how we would take the medicine, and what to do when we took it. Most important was how to lay down and surrender to it in order to work with the medicine and not resist it.

The 5-MeO-DMT is secreted from the Sonoran desert toad. They take the poison from the toad, crystalize it, then you smoke it. It's the same chemical that is released in the brain when you die. It is almost guaranteed you will have a transformational experience when you smoke it no matter the dosage because you experience the same thing that happens in your brain when you die, in some sense.

I didn't know any of that then. I just had a little insight, and I knew it had worked for Mike Tyson. I also knew I didn't have any options, and that it might help me. I was not prepared for what was about to happen.

The guide, Uncle Mike (who looks like a modern-day Big Lebowski), explained that the first dose was a lighter one, an introduction. As you smoke it, within 10 seconds you go into an experience. This lighter dose was to teach me and show me how it works. How to surrender, just let go, and flow through the experience. It showed me that grievances I had did not matter in the grand scheme of things and it connected me to my ancestors in a way I didn't know was possible.

It was also powerful because the healer was played music and sang during the ceremony. He gave you medicine and sang his heart out and played music for you to heal. That combination was very powerful to me and for anyone that I have ever witnessed receive the medicine. It has a breakthrough transformational effect on people's experience and healing process.

After that first dose you have a sense of how things work. The second dose is what they call an individual journey, and it is a much larger dose. And *that* is the one that launches you. I thought I had an idea how it worked after the first one, but it was just enough to get a sensc of what could happen; it shook me and put me into a complete state of awe.

When it was time for the second one, I felt resistance again. I said, "No, I don't need to do another round." I was trying to hold on to my ego, or whatever it was that I was afraid of from before. But, with reassurance and encouragement to maximize my experience, I took that second dose, and it changed my life forever.

The healer counted down from 10. And I just got launched. Completely. That experience was the most powerful, dramatic, tragic thing I've experienced in my life. I experienced a full-on life review.

The best way I can describe it is that I went through a death experience that was very tragic. And in that experience, I saw my life in review and all the key things in my life, including some of the impact that I made on people. Then I got to feel and see that all the seeds I planted throughout my life grew and took off. I saw that everything I was doing was making a difference, and I got to feel that on a very deep level. I also got to feel the tragedy of not being here anymore. And how my family had to live without me. And my work team, and my circle and tribe were all left on their own to do this without me. It put me in touch with my purpose in a way that I could never have imagined.

Everything I saw in my experience was all self-inflicted death. It was a car accident that I created. Going through it was so real. It was the most transformational thing I ever experienced. I remember holding and grasping onto the healer, because I was in such a tragic state and traumatized thinking I was dead. When I was able to get up and walk around, I felt very different.

Before I got up, the healer played music and sang for me. He was doing a warrior's homecoming, everything he could to welcome me home, and welcome me to my new life.

I walked around like a little kid. I smelled the roses that were around me and played in the dirt. There were a bunch of fully grown marijuana plants and I laid down in the middle of them. I didn't believe anything at this point. Nothing was real to me anymore. I didn't believe my car was out front, I did not think I was alive. I was in a different dimension.

This experience broke all those feedback loops and shattered them into a trillion pieces. Everything I was obsessing about, all the things that were dragging me down, depressing me, that I couldn't escape before felt distant as I fully let go of all the things that were not serving me. It shattered everything. It burned everything to the ground. Now here I was at ground zero, square one in life. It was a full reset.

After this second dose, they took us through one more round of the ceremony. This was another small dose, to get me back into my body and ready to move forward. This third dose was like a lot of downloads and information about the path forward for me. A lot of it was about connecting fractured relationships with my family members. Things that had been unacknowledged or dealt with in the back of my mind. Showing me how important it is to face these things, and how I am supposed to show up in the world.

I saw how I was supposed to help others to break through with mental health the same way I had done, and guide others to break through the noise and accept and live their life. A lot of it had to do with mental health. I didn't see it at the time, but when I work with human performance, mental health is a big part of that journey. It was all connected to the stuff I was working on.

After that third dose, I stayed for a while to absorb the experience because things still did not feel real. I took the healer out to dinner that night to express my gratitude. I also needed to see him in a real environment and to start building the layers of reality back. My ego surrendered, and I felt reborn like I was experiencing a new world.

After dinner, rather than staying at the house, I headed toward home. I ended up staying at the same hotel and the same exact room that I stayed at on my way up. Part of me felt like I was in a twilight zone. Part of me felt like a new person, but here I was right where I had stayed before. I questioned what my reality was going to be after this. I was freaked out with the whole thing, but I also felt so transformed. I'm not sure I will ever be able fully explain it.

The next day, I drove home to San Diego. I had my shirt off, I was dancing, I was happy. I hadn't experienced that in so long, I didn't even know what this feeling was.

I felt like I was in a totally different space, and I was in a new chapter in my life. Then when I got home, all these things started to happen. The healer had told me to relisten to some of Mike Tyson's podcasts about the toad and 5-MeO-DMT, because it would give me vocabulary to share with others about this experience. And he told me, "Now that you've had this experience, you will be an ambassador for this medicine and can help others." This was September 9, 2019.

Within two weeks, I was back, and things started to get connected in these crazy ways in life. Synchronicity was showing up. Within two weeks I had all these people tell me that I needed to meet this guy in LA, a Navy SEAL who was going through a lot with his personal life and business and was a few years into his transition. When I connected with him, I looked in his face, and I saw the same stuff I had in myself before I met the healer. I could just tell where he was at emotionally. I kept asking what was wrong. He finally opened up and shared how dark of a place he was in. We barely knew each other, but I could see it because I just went through it. He was the first person I connected with the medicine.

The weekend after I had gone to Northern California, the healer was going to be in town, so I got him connected with the Navy SEAL to do a journey with him. And funny enough, that same guy invited me to a workout and at that workout, I ended up meeting Eben Britton, who has since become a very good friend. Eben worked with Mike Tyson at Tyson Ranch with the podcast. He got all my contact information and invited me to come to Tyson Ranch for a live podcast.

So, there I was, three weeks after this journey and I found myself at Tyson Ranch, taking photos with Mike Tyson. It was surreal. A lot of things like that have happened since I did that journey.

Whether you want to frame it as God, a higher power, or something else, it's learning to surrender to God's plan but also being way more open to seeing the signs that life is showing you. Instead of forcing and trying so hard to run the show, I'm a little more separated from it now, paying more attention and surrendering to what is coming for me, instead of trying to force things to go my way.

Shortly after this, I was at UCLA for a medical follow-up and the doctors couldn't believe what they were seeing. Before I did the 5-MeO-DMT, I was supposed to go for the six-week inpatient Operation Mend program based on my previous assessment. But I had made a full 180° turn. All my assessments were completely opposite from before and they didn't think I needed to do the program anymore. Their minds were blown. Some of my doctors cried because the person I was before was not the same person who was in front of them. They were happy for me but also shocked because they had never seen that happen. I was honest with them about what medicine I did.

Some people look at psychedelics as a taboo topic, like it's a drug or something scary. The thing to understand is that plant medicine is different from pharmaceuticals and human-made drugs. It has its own intelligence. You can't overdose on it. Yes, you can have a bad trip or rough journey if you take too much, but you can't die from overdosing. It's also not addictive. You can use plant medicine to break addiction, but you won't likely get addicted to it. Iboga, another plant medicine in the medicine wheel, is primarily used to cure addictions and help addicts heal and break through.

That said, it is not for everybody, it should be approached with caution and intention. But for some, it can be life-changing or lifesaving. It's taken integration, but my life is better from this experience. I also have not had alcohol since that first journey. I didn't go into it with the intention to stop drinking, but it lost its appeal. The downloads I got told me that alcohol was destroying my quality of life and the lives of people around me. Drinking lowers my vibration and holds my spirit down. I received such clear messages about that, and afterwards, I fully stopped drinking.

Other things improved as well once I completed that first journey. I had issues and fractured relationships everywhere. Issues with neighbors, biological family, many others. After this, I reconnected with my family. My parents and I have an open dialogue now, whereas before I had them blocked and I didn't want to have anything to do with them. I've done a lot of work and forgiven them and want them to have the best and fullest lives possible. I fixed those fractured relationships for myself, which created a lot of healing, and now I don't have any grievances or drama with them.

I've learned that just blocking people doesn't work. The saying, "What you resist, persists," is a major lesson that I have learned, and am still learning. Because it keeps coming up until you deal with it. It's better to approach and lean in to what's bothering you than to avoid it. Sometimes having these conversations are difficult. Sometimes it's magical. When you live fully, you experience the highs and lows.

The way I had compartmentalized certain things had also created a lot of breakdowns, trying to keep things separate or be in a place where I told some people some things, and other people other things. Now I want to just fully be myself 100% of the time.

After the toad ceremony, people started coming into my life who I was able to pay it forward and help provide them with the same opportunity to have a new lease on life. I helped transform their lives by getting them connected to a healer. My network of healers expanded fast, incredible healers who can do work for anyone. I've gotten my whole family—my sister, my aunt, and others—to experience healing in many ways. I've seen countless friends embrace the healing work and witnessed how it helped them move through whatever was haunting them and move forward.

It's not just been a breakthrough for me, but for everyone who is in my circle I share it with. My way of being, or anyone's way of being, creates a ripple effect of impact on anyone who is around them, or who encounters them. I know that the way that I was before this experience created a negative impact around me. Because I was in such a depressed state, it was a ripple effect flowing from me. And even on my toughest days, I want to be in a positive ripple.

Oxygen Mask

Taking action and forcing this hard drive reset changed my life. It also served as a permanent reminder of the importance of taking care of yourself. Taking care of yourself is like keeping your oxygen mask on, as instructed on airplanes. Self-care and regular maintenance, whether physical, emotional, or mental, help you navigate life's challenges. Just like a software update or program hard reset, self-care keeps your systems running efficiently. Design your life so that even on bad days, weeks, or months, you have the resilience to bounce back.

CHAPTER 9

Expansion and Breakthroughs

Healing is a humbling journey and there is no magic fix. It is a mistake to think that the journey is over after you have your first breakthrough toward healing, especially with plant medicines. No matter the methods taken, pre-integration and post-integration are key.

That said, with plant medicine, it's a miracle what can happen when that sacred process unfolds. It's important to remain open to the possibility of life. It shows you how little you know, while clearing the hard drive or resetting yourself. These resets are a reminder that I am a constant white belt in life. It's a reminder that I don't know anything, and I am a beginner.

I had reached max capacity of what I could handle, and I needed a reset. In the military we work with all different kinds of radios and field computers to provide communication in between teams and supporting elements. Sometimes the system gets overloaded and the only way to get the equipment to function again is to hold the off button and do a hard reset. Full shutdown. Reset. Restart. A lot of times this method works. I am reminded of this example because my brain felt like a computer that needed a hard reset.

It's possible to create this reset internally through this work as well as other methods, but it's always important to maintain a beginner's mindset.

When looking at Eastern versus Western medicine it's important to understand the programing and brainwashing that's occurred in the name of pharmaceuticals, money, power, and control. There have been massive campaigns spreading the belief and labels that plant medicines are dangerous or hippie drugs. It is disrespectful to label them like that, especially after what I've witnessed over the last few years, from my own experience, and seeing the impact on people I know and their families. There is a fear of the unknown, and people often have conscious or unconscious fear of something because it is foreign to them. These are some of the trappings that come with living in a comfort zone of someone else's construction.

That said, and I cannot stress this enough, educating yourself on the process of using plant medicines and planning are key. I have heard of bad instances, like individuals doing it in an uncontrolled setting and having an adverse reaction. Someone who has a severe personality disorder should not take a plant medicine psychedelic by themselves; without some type of integration plan it can be dangerous.

With psychedelics, and plant medicine in particular, there is a medicine wheel of different plants that can help heal every part of us when approached thoughtfully with intention, even later in life.

There is a 70+-year-old man I know with a heart condition who started with something very low key like a psilocybin chocolate that created a heart-opening experience. It was transformational for him. I've also seen somebody in their late 80s go from having severe dementia to seeing positive effects after microdosing psilocybin. He has seen noticeable improvement of cognitive function and speech, and his overall life engagement went way up. And that's my grandfather, Papa. To see his shift in mood and happiness has been incredible.

Many different friends from the military have experienced a powerful, even magical, warrior's homecoming through plant medicine and integration work. Connecting others into the healing work has become very meaningful to me, considering the journey I know so many have gone through, and the struggles that come from their experiences and how they frame and attach to those experiences.

All of the healing circles I have been privileged to sit in have been different and had their own healing qualities and downloads/takeaways. Some of them were accomplished through psilocybin, 5-MeO-DMT, ayahuasca, or cactus—medicines where you don't have to do anything except set an intention, but you can have truly transformational experiences that become a gateway to a lot of healing.

My first toad journey was one of the most sacred and powerful experiences I've ever had in my entire life. It was September 9, 2019. I was 35 at that time. And I have not had a sip of alcohol since then.

I didn't know what I was getting into but I am so grateful that it happened. I had the best kind of guide, somebody who was extremely caring, with a love for former military guys, and who loves to do these homecoming warrior circles.

Going into it, I didn't have an intention—and as I had been having suicidal thoughts, I was genuinely at the end of my rope. I was saying I didn't want to be alive anymore, and that I was done with life. I was at full capacity. The only intention I had was to try and get some sort of reset.

Before the first healing ceremony, I felt like I was in some cookie-cutter life that I did not recognize, like in the *Matrix*. I didn't have an intention set for the experience, like I would today. I simply needed to reset, and that served as my intention. And I did get a reset. And through that experience, I got scared straight but I knew that I definitely wanted to live.

I always advise seeking medical guidance and following a system or process if you are considering a plant medicine healing journey, and that you do as much research as possible. First and foremost, research and vet the healer or group that you are considering doing this with. There are some people serving plant medicines who do not have good intentions or the experience that qualifies them to guide you in a healing way or hold the proper space. I include a simple checklist of key terms that a reputable healer/guide will use in the Resources section of my website.

Awareness about plant medicine is growing every day. Former special operations veterans and other trauma survivors are finally getting the breakthroughs they need after the failure of so many other methods of medicine. This is going to continue to expand and there will be more and more use of these medicines for veterans and civilians to combat post-traumatic stress and depression.

As these modalities gain in popularity and approval through decriminalization, legalization, and research studies, especially in the veteran community, it's opening the gates and more people are getting into it. It's also more important than ever to share the sacred knowledge and science behind what it is, and to help set proper expectations.

In big healing sessions, typically there are healers or watchers who support everybody in the ceremony. They hold the space to heal and work through whatever you need to work through. These individuals play a very critical role.

One significant point is not to do this on your own. Where you do it, how you do it, and whom you have around you is extremely important. Talk to people in your circle or somebody who has had the experience. Keep in mind, everyone's experience is different, but you can set yourself up for success with the medicine you are trying and for the ceremony by researching and learning from others.

Thankfully, I have a great community around me, and as I began to integrate my experiences, and share about them with my community, I began to let go and move forward. A strong community is medicine and with a strong circle you can bounce back from anything.

Circle of Trust

For me, trust is always an obstacle and has been for my whole life, so having a circle of trust is a big part of my growth: being able to open up to others and build trust and relationships. The basis of the culture in the community for us at Deep End Fitness (DEF) and Underwater Torpedo League starts with a circle of trust.

To begin and end every session, we form a circle, go around the circle and say who we are, why we are there, and what our goals are for this session. Following the session, we repeat this process, sharing our takeaways. This protocol creates a trustful environment. It is a vulnerable situation for humans to go underwater, and this creates a lot of authenticity and a powerful community and connection throughout the training experience.

Since we started DEF, I don't know how many sessions I have led—hundreds on hundreds of sessions where I've been in circles of trust at the beginning and end of every session. This practice of being vulnerable and opening up to each other creates a lot of growth for me and for others. I have worked with and learned from thousands of individuals, and have identified patterns that apply to human performance, unlocking potential in all areas of life, not just in the pool.

This has also brought a sense of self-actualization and acceptance. Being in a leadership role within the community, I have constantly pushed myself (and been pushed and stretched) outside of my comfort zone, to push and grow the community, programs, and drive the dream forward. It has stretched me so far. I find myself in constant amazement. Part of me resists the titles. I don't want a title at this point. But when it comes to my role, it comes with a set of obstacles and challenges to overcome as we create something completely new and scale it worldwide. There are growing pains as we test and learn to find the way. This mission has been a huge catalyst for growth for Don, Ricky, me, and our entire team, including all our amazing instructors who continue to level up.

It has been incredible working with extraordinary humans. From the professional athletes, Olympic athletes, challenged athletes, or even athletes of high caliber who don't know how to swim, I have gotten to see a lot of different scenarios and learn from all of them. I like working with all types of individuals at this point, not just athletes. To see the leaps of confidence added to people's lives and be able to contribute to them has really made an impact on me and means so much.

On top of the immense purpose that contributing gives me, it's so inspiring to work with all these professional athletes and see the commitment and effort they put into their crafts. I grew up watching all types of sports and pro athletes on TV, and now I get to work with some of the top athletes from many different sports.

It is purposeful working with these athletes, not just in sports performance, but supporting them in unlocking potential in all aspects of life. Each time I see their performance grow in the pool

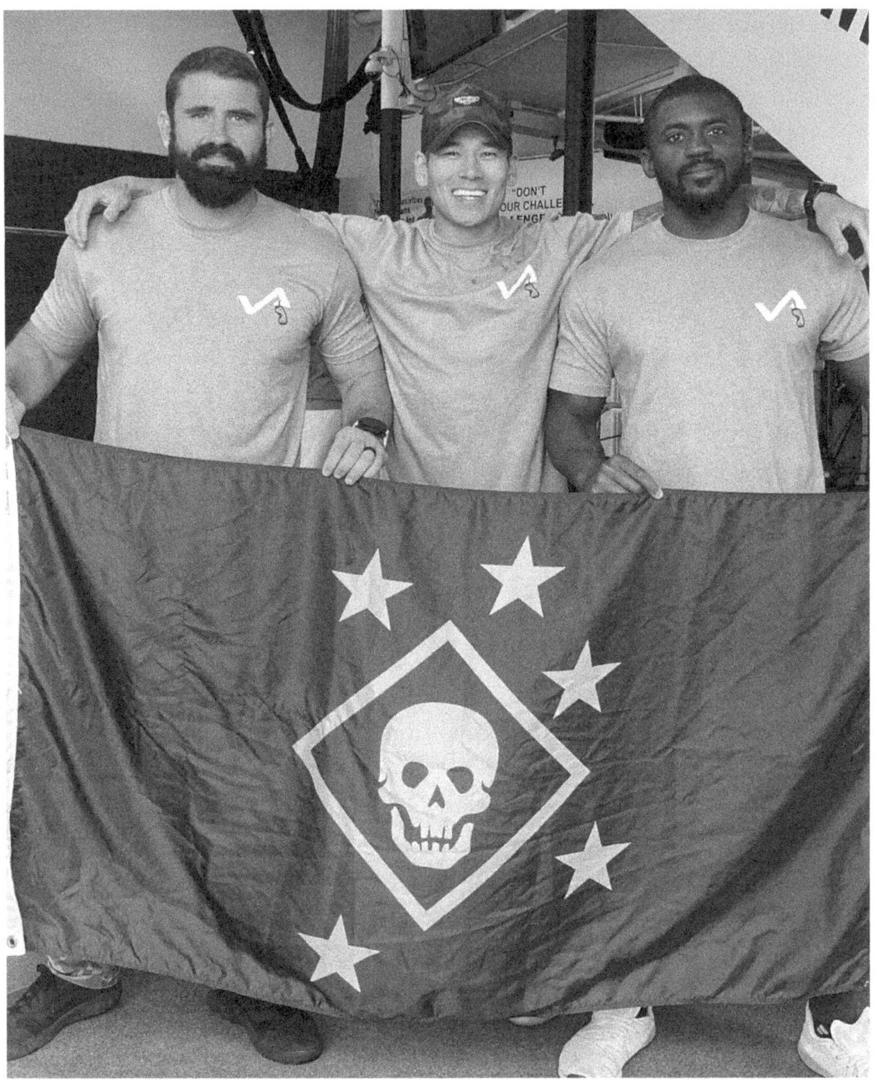

Prime with Marine Raider brothers Don Tran and Ricky after a Memorial Day event in California, in 2024

and in life, I grow as a coach, and the programs grow. But being able to work with people who are some of the best in the world at what they do and help them grow and transform their lives is very special.

Another thing that's been a constant since getting out of the marines is working with young men and women going into the military, to mentor and help them. I find a lot of purpose in this work because I get to give them what I missed when I went into the military. I focus on giving them the real information, taking a hard look at their life and situation with them, and supporting their preparation, being a guide and helping them understand and define their why. At a minimum, by the time they go in, they have a strong reason why they are enlisting.

My default answer to anyone who wants to join the military is that I never recommend going in at all. I ask what other options or skills they have so they do not need to join. If the candidates that are persistent, I continue to ask, "Why do you want this?" and "Why?" and "Why?" until they can prove to me and themselves with a strong enough reason for why they want to go in before I agree to work with them.

I've also had a lot of experience working with transitioning military. I know firsthand that transitioning can be a hard fight. Leaving your identity behind is challenging. As I've mentioned, it's easy to become institutionalized in the military. Sometimes it feels like you are on an island or in a vacuum within society. You're used to getting paid every two weeks; your identity is tied to your job, rank, and so on; and then one day, you must give it all up. You have to be able to let all that go from your life. At first it can be daunting to fill your entire hierarchy of needs and not have the military to support you. I know just how hard that can be, and I am committed to being a part of the solution.

I have had a lot of opportunities to develop systems and processes from pattern recognition that I've unlocked from working with different individuals, groups, and teams. I'm grateful for the opportunities that I get to mentor others and work in the capacity as a human performance and transformational coach. The impact I get to make helps bring everything full circle. One of the things that brings me the most joy in life is supporting others in unlocking their goals.

Culture Shifts

When I was finishing my undergraduate degree, I wrote one of my final papers about culture. I realized that you can't just change culture overnight. You can't just decide to change it and make all these hard changes just happen at once.

However, what you can do is create shifts. These shifts can add up to waves of change. So, every day, my mission is to create these shifts to make the world a better place, as much as I can, as much as my organization can. This starts with making sure my oxygen mask is on and that I'm continuing to heal and integrate.

A lot of times, how that shows up is having hard conversations with people. I've learned to set boundaries with people who are toxic or create cancer (culture vultures and energy vampires) because we cannot make a positive shift if we have that in the culture. It's not always rainbows and unicorns. It's having real conversations that create authentic relationships. It's important to be open and honest with ourselves and with others about how we are showing up. These boundaries are necessary so that I, or we as an organization, have the most bandwidth and ability to unlock a positive shift in others.

Unlocking a state of flow also requires making daily shifts in my own life with the resources that I have available to me, which is one lesson that came out from training all these athletes, especially the fighters. Being in Southern California, we are fortunate there a some of the best martial arts training for jiu jitsu, grappling, kickboxing, mixed martial arts, boxing, and so on in the United States and in the world.

Some of the fighters have plugged me in with the right coaches, and over the last few years, I have expanded myself with martial arts training. I started off in a crawling phase. Learning the techniques and moves, building combinations with punches, then eventually kicks. Then I eventually added jiu jitsu and groundwork, then into sparring. All of that has been a process of self-actualization and inner work to heal and evolve.

For years, I drove by these places thinking, *Oh man, I wish I could do that.* But then I started to shift my thoughts to *Why not? Why can't I do this?* I now live more fully and go after the things that interest me or I feel called to explore.

Now I have confidence to go into these places, try something new, or work to get better at. I join classes or get private training or sessions. This has influenced every aspect of my life positively. The beautiful thing is most of us can apply this to any goal we have or hobby we have been meaning to start. Intention, consistency, and support/accountability systems are great ingredients to make anything happen!

Focus on Where You Want to Go

When you try new things, it can be a confidence builder, and you start to think about what else you can do that you might have been hesitant to try before. For instance, I always wanted to learn how to surf. Along our training and coaching journey, I've had the opportunity to work with and train pro surfers, including Cole Houshmand, and now he's my coach, too. He trains me on the same waves he trained on with his dad, Shawn Houshmand, for over 20 years. They take me and push me, and I've gained some new skills, but even more important confidence and joy. Now I get to see Cole crushing the pro tour and winning competitions like Rip Curl Pro at Bells Beach, Australia. He competes at the highest levels. I learned from working with Cole and Shawn to "focus on where you want to go," which means literally stare at the direction and area that you want your surfboard to move in, and it works every time. If I look up or down, I wipe out, but when I lock in and stare at the right side of the wave, I find that I move exactly where I want to go. I feel that this can be applied to so much in life.

When we worked with the US Ski and Snowboard Team, we learned they also follow this principle (Note: Alpine skiers on the US Ski and Snowboard Team can reach speeds of over 80 miles per hour in downhill and super-G races). The athletes and coaches explained that the one thing they can never do in a race is focus on the obstacles. Instead, they focus on the open area that they want to move toward or cover. This is a high stakes form of "focus on where you want to go" and a reminder to be mindful of what you put your focus on.

We all have things that hold us back from trying new things. Money was something that used to hold me back. But now my relationship with money has changed. This applies also to receiving. I used to not charge for training sometimes or do coaching for free and not accept payment even when people offered. Now I have evolved to be able to accept and receive more. I realize money is important to continue to make a greater impact.

While money is important to me, what matters to me most is my relationships and my network. I find that when I prioritize them, everything turns out to be reciprocal in some sense. That has shown up for me in the different experiences that I have received, by giving to others.

It is amazing how underwater training affects your performance. I've seen it over and over in others. But it's been key for me in finding ways to grow and develop myself as well. These experiences have helped me unlock my full creativity and flow state and ultimately help me be the best version of myself that I can be.

After seeing all of the results from 15 years of underwater training and witnessing incredible breakthroughs, we pursued a research study in 2021 that was published by *Frontiers*, and which was led by our team's neuroscientist, Dr. William (Jamie) Tyler.

The study was designed to be a four- to six-week study on a cohort of 60 athletes who attended a minimum of one DEF pool session per week across the experimental time frame. We measured mental performance markers before and after DEF exposure.

The results were incredible:

- DEF significantly reduces stress (by 27.1%).
- DEF significantly reduces anxiety (by 32.6%).
- In a study of 40 experimental subjects, 56% saw improvements in depression and 63% saw improvements in anxiety and stress (compared to pharmaceuticals/antidepressants/ selective serotonin reuptake inhibitors, which claim to have a success rate between 50% and 75%).

These breakthroughs happen so rapidly for our athletes because when you are underwater, a survival response goes off in your mind, which can put you into a panic state if not managed, so this is why we train to manage mental focus and be able to relax on demand.

This goes back to our key framework of F.R.E.E.: focus, relaxation, economy of motion, efficient breathing.

When you go underwater and get into this survival state, you can also learn about yourself and what is stressing you out. Sometimes you never know what's going to come to the surface. You might get some crazy thoughts when you are underwater. You have to focus and face them.

Things come up if you have too much going on, or something bothering you that you can't block out; it can be hard to close those mental tabs. Once you get into the habit of decluttering your mind, then it becomes easier to be underwater and perform at a high level.

We are finding more and more that when you put yourself in that underwater environment, safely exposing yourself for longer periods of time, it can help you evolve coping mechanisms. You can approach your feelings and problems instead of avoiding them. This is approached-based coping. It becomes easier to override doing something challenging when you master controlling your mind in an uncomfortable environment, and it becomes easier to do hard things. Rather than when you are avoiding your problems, now you are trying to resist. Resisting is like trying to put your hand over a faucet that is blasting water or swimming upstream against a current.

Do you approach or avoid your problems? The more you approach them, and stare down that fear, we realize that a lot of things our minds make are illusions. But the more you lean in and face it, the more that stuff just disappears, and your performance continues to improve.

Sometimes you need to move toward your resistance in life. Run toward the gunfire, even though that seemingly doesn't make sense. Move toward your biggest fear. Go underwater. Go swim if you have never swam before. Next time you see a loved one, stretch yourself to go one step deeper in connecting with them. All those things are approach versus avoid.

My personal example was fearing heights from my early fall off the roof and fracturing my skull. This held me back from trying different things. When I went into special operations, I had to get my skydiving qualifications. I had to face my fear of heights by parachuting, freefalling, and even the low-level static line jumps especially those in which we got to land in the ocean. Eventually facing and overcoming this fear unlocked a new confidence for me to do other things; for example, going on a tall ladder no longer bothers me.

In special operations training, if I had gone to the edge of the aircraft, stopped, and said, "I can't do this," and quit, that would have been the end of my progress and growth. It's key in these moments when we want to quit to face our obstacles and move through our fears and resistance toward personal freedom.

The third principle of the F.R.E.E. system is economy of motion. This requires understanding the concepts of flow and drag. The two biomechanics of swimming are increased propulsion and reduced friction. This simply means adding flow and eliminating drag. Any bad or extra movement, in swimming, driving, or anything you are doing in life that requires movement, prevents our highest performance. Why does this matter? The inefficient movements add up, the drag adds up, holding us back, limiting us from our highest potential in whatever we are doing.

How can we eliminate drag? It's easy to identify the physical, but how do you identify mental or emotional drag? The most surefire way is to notice when you have resistance to something.

At first, you might not understand what drag or where resistance shows up. This can occur in the form of a challenging moment, fight or flight, or feeling like you don't want to do something.

It's not always easy to see when drag is holding us back from flow. This is one of the reasons that mentors and coaches are so important for personal growth. I have found that to show up as my best, I need to ensure that I have mentors, training partners, and mentees. These are great accountability systems to stay on track or continue moving forward in the direction that you want to go.

- ◆ **Mentors:** Learn from the previous generations who have been successful and now are in a position to give back and share information to keep paying it forward.
- ◆ **Training partners:** These are people on the same level playing field in life, business, and so on. These are trusted individuals you can train and spar with, and also bounce ideas off and learn and grow through experience.
- ◆ **Mentees:** These are younger or up-and-coming individuals seeking information and guidance whom you can work with and give back to and support. For me, it's working with kids going into the military or athletes who are trying to break through to the next level. It's valuable to them and for me to have a chance to be what's missing for them in their lives.

Expansion Takes a Village

I want to give special recognition to the people who have really made an impact on me, including my mentors, training partners, and mentees. And, to my family. The growth and expansion I've experienced wouldn't be possible without them.

My kids have enabled some of my best expansion. My daughter Hanna Joy, my grandmother's namesake, has unlocked new levels of joy in my life. Joy is something I missed a lot throughout my life. It's very special to me that my daughter shares the same name as my grandmother. My daughter has a very fun personality, she's super funny, sometimes likes to play tricks on people, and brings so much delight to everyone in our house.

My son Trey is the most focused kid who just wants to help everyone as much as possible. Since he was in fifth grade, he has been running laps around our neighborhood and will run up to 6 miles a week as an extra conditioning tool for his sports. Trey also does jiu jitsu a couple times a week, is a quarterback for his football team, plays soccer, and does underwater training. He has two-a-days almost every day. At his middle school he runs in the annual jogathon, where the kids run as many laps as possible in an hour. He clocked over 6 miles in an hour. He has also run two half-marathons. He ran his first half when he was eight years old. Now he runs a sub-six-minute mile. Trey is a very intelligent and helpful person to have around and pushes everyone around him to do their best.

My wife Brittany is a powerhouse. She is the Executive Director of PrimeHall.com, managing all of my speaking and training events. She also has consulting company, Refraem, and *always* has impressive performance; no matter what she does or what company she works with, she excels. She does the workload of 10 capable people. It is just amazing to see what she's working on, not to mention everything she does for our family and those in our community.

Our home is full of crazy performers. Between Brittany and me, we foster a high-performing environment, and the kids seem to feed off it. We have two dogs, an English bulldog, and a Frenchie. A bigger dog and smaller dog is a fun dynamic. Having them around enhances the quality of life and supports our emotional and mental health and overall well-being.

And I love my team; getting to work with Don and Ricky is a huge blessing. We have gone through a lot over the years, from our time in the military together and in business. We've gone through some of the highest highs and lowest of lows. I just appreciate them more than words can express for continuing to ride *everything* with me and continuously evolving and growing. Our team continues to grow.

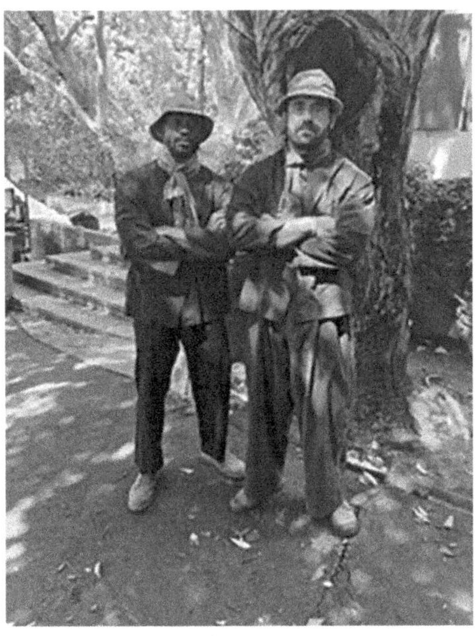

Prime and Ricky (2018)

A lot of the obstacles I have experienced have created huge opportunities along the way, and through these opportunities I have created a powerful network of warrior-minded people, who all have this common thread of wanting to make this world a better place and who strive to perform better, evolve and grow to be better in a merit-based environment. Everyone wants to learn and then give it to others, so they can also unlock results. This unlocks a powerful ripple effect.

CHAPTER 10

Self-Realization

You can design a life that prioritizes growth, authenticity, and meaningful relationships while clearing the noise that distracts from your purpose. The deeper you go within, the more empowered and free from resistance you become, ensuring you are set up to live your life in flow. It isn't about avoiding challenges or obstacles but about navigating them intentionally.

Sometimes the only way to the other side of an obstacle is straight through. My sobriety from alcohol and prescription medications has been a deep journey filled with highs and lows. As I've mentioned, when I got out of the marines, I was put on all the medications. Within a year of getting out, I suffered from many of the side effects that came with them. I started transitioning away from taking these meds. I had started my master of business administration program, and I was taking CBD and herbs for pain relief, headaches, and migraines. I still felt like I needed something to help mask my social anxiety, so I started drinking again after 10 years of sobriety. My excuse at the time was how long I had gone without drinking, so I gave myself permission to drink. But I soon found myself drinking more and more. I thought that alcohol masked my problems, but it became a tool and coping strategy to avoid my problems.

So here I was fresh out of the military, drinking again, and over-doing it. At the same time, I was diving into human performance and studying patterns in the athletes I worked with to better understand what was working and not working for them, and how to level up in any area. I coached these amazing athletes and witnessed their discipline. This led me to look at myself and ask questions about my own life choices.

When I did drink, it's like it unlocked a superhighway to all the things that bothered me. I would go into a victim mindset, and feelings of survivor's guilt moved to the surface. I experienced intrusive thoughts and emotions, anger stemming from childhood to endless questioning about why I was still here while lost their lives either in combat or on returning home and not being able to cope with the transitions or aftermath of their time at war.

The discipline I saw in the athletes I worked with who were training to compete in sports like the Ultimate Fighting Championship (UFC), NFL, or the Olympics forced me to look even deeper at the patterns in myself. I became more and more aware that drinking did not work for me. With a family history of alcoholism, it was a pattern I had seen in others my whole life. Plus, I knew it had gotten me in a lot of trouble previously. I knew that I perform better in everything and I have more peace when I am not drinking. I'd proven that before. Alcohol is a depressant, and if you have negative feedback loops like I did, when you throw alcohol into the equation, it can magnify the negative feedback loops and enhance and feed the depression.

And, as I've mentioned, by the time I made it to my first healing journey with 5-MeO-DMT, I was at the very end of my rope with my mental health and being able to cope. I did not have a clear intention to stop drinking, but one of the things that came from smoking the toad venom that day is that I never wanted to drink again. I saw how alcohol was killing me and everyone around me was suffering from it. It's hard to put into words how impactful sobriety from alcohol has been for me. That one healing experience unlocked a positive change that has lasted to this day. I still don't have any desire to drink alcohol.

With the self-realizations that I had about my relationship with alcohol, combined with the experience of the healing ceremony, it almost became effortless to let go of drinking alcohol. This helped me instantly unlock new levels of performance. I saw improvements in my focus, breathing, and relaxation. It gave me the space and opportunity to figure out how to deal with some of the challenging situations and memories. I started to crack codes to the problems I was working through and my quality of life improved.

When in Doubt, Focus Out

A lot of times when I am dealing with stressful situations, or my mental health or emotional health is challenged, I do my best to focus outwards on something or someone external I can support and make a positive difference for. One of my best friends Dom Cruz always tells me, "When in doubt, focus out."

Learning how to focus outwards is important, yet sometimes you need to lean in. While in the military, I felt like a robot. I was in a checklist mentality and there was no room to dwell in my emotions. After getting out and going through transition, then doing a lot of healing work, I now had more access to my emotions. I can feel things that I couldn't necessarily feel before, which can be uncomfortable. Through this discomfort I learned that it's important to lean in instead of avoiding it when there's something uncomfortable, especially emotionally.

As you approach and deal with your problems, you can begin to move past them. When you avoid them, they will creep up and start to circle and haunt you.

Choosing to be sober from alcohol has given me the ability to build a strong foundation for mental, emotional, spiritual, and psychological health. I now have minimal problems or negative things in my life. When I was not sober and drinking all the time, I was in a clouded mindset, and I had all types of problems and issues with my relationships. Many of my connections with others were inauthentic or full of friction. An unhealthy version of my ego was quick to show up.

Since my healing journey began, I have had realizations and self-actualized them. Now, I'm growing all my key relationships and working on myself and looking for any way that I can support others in my circle or in my life. Most of the problems that I have personally are logistical things that our team is working on solving at work. Our team is constantly growing and with growth comes growing pains. It's crazy to look back and see how much we all have evolved individually and collectively since we started. It's surreal to see how big the community has become, and also the potential for future growth is massive.

Sometimes I think back to the problems we had in Afghanistan, which were extreme life or death, and compare it to some stressor we are dealing with in the company or some drama over an email, or whatever the case may be. These are first-world problems and are good problems to have; it's ultimately rewarding to see them play out.

Overcoming Victim Mindset

Before I started my path to healing, during my medical separation from the military, I was going to nonstop appointments, and I was asked so many questions. The doctors asked me about my experiences, how I dealt with my trauma and Post-Traumatic Stress. I tried not to take on the victim mindset; however, I did fall into this mindset shortly into my transition. This led me into some dark times. What I was resisting was persisting.

My victim mindset wasn't just from the military; it was also childhood. My flashbacks started to happen frequently when my son was the age I had been when I had my most traumatic experiences. I also found myself questioning why or how I made it alive from the experiences in war, and I lived with a lot of survivor guilt. One of the main lessons I learned from this period is that taking control and accountability for whatever happens or fails to happen is *always* the better option over blaming others and asking, *Why me?* Instead, ask *Why not me?* We should always want to take accountability for anything that is in our lives and not be a victim because a victim mindset can kill you.

I'm also grateful for having lived through the experience of having a victim mindset. Yes, this mindset allowed me to hit rock bottom and almost completely break down. But the breakdowns have unlocked so much growth and opportunity for me and my mental health. Each breakdown has ultimately enabled me to reframe the challenges into positives.

At one point, I participated in a monthly working group/workshop focused on human performance for special operations units and professional athletes and teams. In one of these group sessions, I heard about the book by Bruce Schneider, *Energy Leadership: The 7 Level Framework for Mastery in Life and Business* (Wiley, 2022). It helped me think about victim mindsets in a new way. All our thoughts influence our beliefs and actions and shape how we live our lives. I think about what is called *source energy*, and how we're the source of everything in our lives, which starts as our thoughts. *Energy Leadership* shares the following seven-level framework where having the victim mindset is the lowest level that you need to work up from.

Level 1: Victim—I lose.

Level 2: Conflict—You lose.

Level 3: Responsibility—I win.

Level 4: Concern—You win.

Level 5: Opportunity—We both win.

Level 6: Synthesis—All we do is win.

Level 7: Nonjudgmental—Winning and losing is an illusion.

Reframing

First and foremost, since I have learned to put my trust in God's divine plan for me and the world, I have refocused my life toward operating in the light when called to do so.

I've learned how important it is to have a positive approach to framing and adaptive capacity to shift and reframe as much as possible for my own mental health and everyone around me.

For example, the peeping Tom in my window was like a boogeyman who haunted my life and my memories for so long. Now, that memory doesn't haunt me anymore and I have found a way to be grateful for it and realize that it shaped me. I know how to reframe, and now I'm able to look at obstacles and find opportunities or silver linings. That experience gave me a different level of resilience, one that I have been able to use through other challenges.

If I had not had those experiences, I may not have built the resilience I needed that got me through other situations I've been through. I was able to work through those new challenges because I had such a difficult time growing up. I keep realizing more and more that it's all in how you view and process each challenging person, place, thing, or event, and how you frame it. The most powerful way for me to frame it now is that the experience that I had with my peeping Tom was my special ops military training starting early. That experience unlocked so much for me that I was able to tap into it for the rest of my life. If I even saw that guy today, I would not attack him.

Sobriety has been an opportunity to work through these deep-rooted issues. It has provided time and space to heal and the ability to access and lean into traumas that were buried deep in my subconscious, unconscious, and memory bank. A lot of time traumas are buried so deep and it is easy to keep those things buried. But to dig them up and face them creates an opportunity to improve yourself as a whole, including your physical, mental, and emotional health. Doing this can unlock even more healing.

For anyone who is currently battling with mental health I recommend using the building block approach that we use for pool training, which is a simple process that can be applied to learning any new skill. The system I use is crawl, walk, run, fly.

When I stopped drinking and committed to a major lifestyle change, those early days were some of the hardest. I was learning to crawl. The first day, the first week, even the first month of sobriety facing social environments felt like a battle. Drinking had been a mask to hide my anxiety. It was tough to let that go, and I realized how important it was to first make a commitment to myself. Then I could share it with the people I love and trust, those who could help hold me accountable. Having support in my corner made all the difference when things got tough.

Humans are so resilient, adaptable, and capable of making huge changes. You just start with crawling and focus on one day at a time. Focus on the foundation and you will start to feel better. It gets easier with time. Before you know it, two weeks will have passed and then a month, then six months. You will start to see benefits quicker than you might think. You begin to walk, run, then fly.

Living with Traumatic Brain Injury (TBI)

When I was eight, I experienced my first TBI when I fractured my skull. I had additional trauma to my brain throughout life with car accidents, getting beaten up badly, having bottles cracked over my head, the explosions in the insider attack, concussions, and so on.

One of the instances was right before I left for marine boot camp. I was jumped by a group of bouncers at a club. They had assaulted one of the guys I was with after he successfully pissed them off. Turns out these bouncers had a pattern of doing this to marines leaving for boot camp. They would look for and target them. The situation that night escalated and turned into a group fight between myself and my drunk friend and the bouncers. But he ran away as soon as he could. So, it really was me versus the bouncers until things got bloody. There were 10–15 bouncers on the site at the club. Only about half of them jumped me, taking turns kicking me while I was on the ground. Sometimes it was more of a one-on-one situation.

The bouncers would not fight me if I moved off the club property, so I stepped out of the parking lot to get a breather. Then my adrenaline kicked back in, I stepped back onto the property, and reengaged the fight, until somebody came up behind me and cracked a bottle on the back of my head. Blood just poured down my head to the point I could throw fistfuls of blood toward the guy who hit me. I had been hit and kicked in the head leading up to this, but this was a serious blow that left me with a concussion and open head wound. The guy who initially started fighting with the bouncers ended up having his orbital bones crushed. We were all beat up pretty badly and supposed to leave for boot camp the next day. It was almost 2:00 a.m. when the fighting ended. We had to arrive to get checked in at boot camp about 4:00 or 5:00 a.m. and we were not in good shape. I had even lost a shoe and had to get a new one, not to mention my head wound. I was not allowed into boot camp because I had an open head wound. They were going to look into what happened and they wouldn't allow me to start until they knew more.

I thought there was no way they would send me to boot camp again and that had been my only chance. I was really upset and thought I would have to do a walk of shame home since my family had already thrown me a going-away dinner and I'd felt their support and pride in my decision to pursue the Marine Corps. But the guy who had his orbital bones broken was able to clear the events up and clear my name of any trouble. The recruiters ended up being super cool with me, and I was able to go again.

About the time I began to write this book, I had a concussion, which put me into a bad mental state. I stayed inside and in dark rooms a lot, hardly going outdoors or in nature so that I could avoid brightness and keep my headaches at bay. It was after sifting through that aftermath that I came up with the rough outline for this book.

I was in such a state that it unlocked certain parts of my brain. I now was able to sit down and get my thoughts for this book organized in a new way. This got me curious about situations where people who have some type of brain injury unlock something incredible because of the injury, like a sudden savant syndrome. There have been cases of post-concussion individuals unlocking mastery levels in math and music.

Even looking back at different traumatic events, those experiences ultimately put me into a new place where I have deeper connections in my life. I have more depth with people and in my relationships, and with things that I do. Before I had a lot of this trauma I felt like I was living on the surface. I'd lie on the couch, watching TV and movies. Not a lot of deep connections and relationships.

These days, instead of having TVs in every room of the house, we have one TV that we let our kids watch. And maybe we'll watch sports when we have an athlete competing, or UFC fights. It's fun for me to watch UFC not only because I like the sport and a lot of the athletes but I also get to watch one of my best friends, Dominick Cruz, commentating the fights most of the time, which is a cool addition to the mix and a reason to tune in.

Otherwise, the general lack of TVs enables me to focus on building deep connections and relationships with my family, my work team, friends, community, and important people, and giving myself space. I'm not able to live on the surface anymore, and I have more focus on depth and connection.

Connection takes being intentional because it's not always pleasant for me to participate in certain activities or be in certain environments, especially when there may be sensory overload with lights and noise.

Going to a restaurant for someone's birthday or to meet a friend can be stressful, especially places with bars, loud music, bright lights, and a lot of people. For some people, it's a walk in the park; for me it's a huge energy drainer. Migraines are easily triggered for me whenever there are a million different sounds. Ultimately, these places are not healthy for me.

Yet, despite the challenges of these situations, when I get myself out of my comfort zone in social environments it unlocks new levels of social resilience.

It also presents an opportunity for me to explain to other people why it's like this for me and share my story. As somebody who likes to make other people around me happy and show up for them, sometimes it requires me to set boundaries for situations that are just not healthy for me, which helps me show up as the best I can.

It is funny looking at what I enjoy or find entertaining now versus when I was younger. I couldn't have imagined myself meditating or seeking quiet places in nature becoming such a priority in my life. But making these choices and changes and communicating about them has led to amazing relationships and experiences that I would never have otherwise.

One day I was in San Diego coaching at one of the pools and pro fighter Dominick Cruz came into a session with some other fighters. He ended up getting hooked on the training; he worked with us a lot and we started hanging out. Over the years, he has become one of my best friends and he's a great influence. He always pushes me to unlock the next levels of performance and challenges me to analyze the way I think about things. I've gained so much perspective from doing personal development courses and emotional intelligence work, all of which has been a game changer for me thanks to Dom. He always shares resources and information. He got me turned on to stem cell therapy, which has fully addressed the extreme back pain I had for years. We talk about the balance in life and how sometimes you are the hammer in life, and sometimes you are the nail. He reminds me that you must train your mind to be ready for both.

With the hammer and nail, it's like losing and winning. It's okay to lose a round here and there and even a fight, but you can never give up.

I learned this in Marine Raider training when I was one of the slower runners and came in nearly last on three- to five-mile runs. It humbled me nearly every morning to start my day with a loss, but I had to be able to let it go and not let it mess up my performance for the rest of the day.

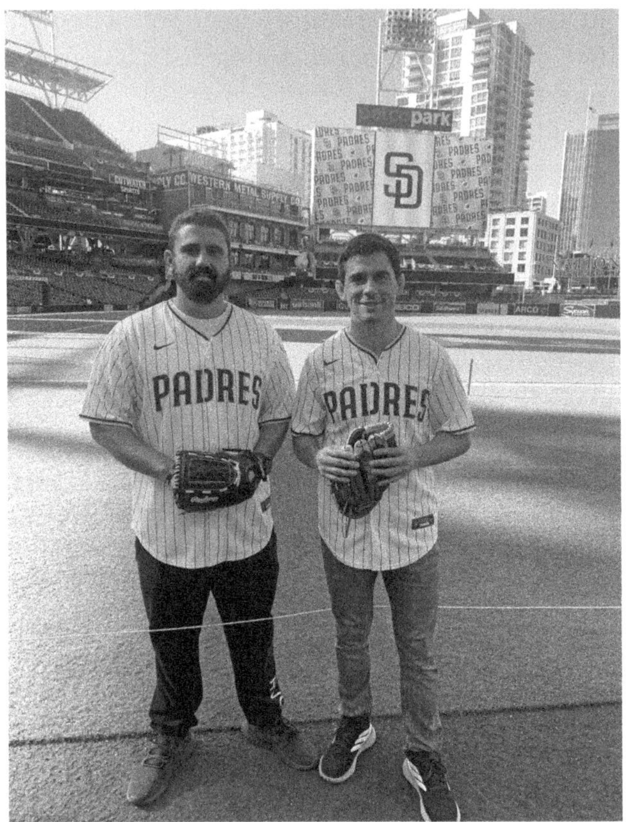

Prime with His Close Friend Dom Cruz Throwing the First Pitch at a Padres Game (2021)

Learning from Toxic Relationships

Since we started our entrepreneurial journey in business, we have had a lot of experiences to learn from. We've been fortunate to have a lot of mentors and support. We'd never started a sport or a company before so naturally we've hit a lot of obstacles as we've been growing that we have had to figure out. And sometimes people see the momentum and growth and want to be part of it. Sometimes for the right reasons, but sometimes not.

We've poured everything into Deep End Fitness (DEF) and Underwater Torpedo League (UTL), including life savings and thousands on thousands of hours of effort, intention, and energy. That makes it especially hurtful and personal when people try to take advantage.

But again, there is always an opportunity—we've learned so much from those experiences. It's sharpened us and turned us more into professionals, we can set ourselves up for success so that those situations don't happen. We've had a lot of growth through those challenges. Business can bring out the best and worst in humanity.

Sometimes growing a business feels like levels in a video game. You've got to learn from the early levels so that you will have the skill and the will to make it through the difficult levels. We have a massive community of supporters who create a massive why for us to continue to grow DEF and UTL. Each obstacle in business and in life seems to come with lessons or a download of information that can be extremely valuable in ensuring that the lessons are learned and not repeated over and over.

Imagine you are kayaking down a white water rapid and you suddenly you hit a huge rock. The rock does slight damage to your kayak but it's still good to continue. What do you do at this point? Do you just continue and hope you don't hit another rock? Or do you create a solution or game plan to mitigate hitting rocks along the route? Any plan is better than no plan.

The question becomes, are we going to zigzag? Or are we going to fly a drone overhead so we know where the rocks are? Any time we hit an obstacle or a failure, it's an opportunity to pivot.

It's been surreal to see how DEF and UTL have grown, especially after keeping the business alive during COVID when almost all our pools shut down. Don and I have put everything into the companies to get to this point. It means a lot to see the traction and growth as DEF and UTL are now growing across the globe. The positive feedback we receive from community members across the United States about the impact that DEF and UTL has had on their lives is one of the greatest rewards of this work.

Depressive Thoughts and Pattern Interrupts

I never want to downplay how challenging depression can be to deal with or give false hope or expectations that there is some magical solution.

When I became aware of my depressive thoughts, I started to notice patterns. I don't know how long I'd had those negative thoughts circling in my mind. It was not constant and seems to have come in and out throughout my life. But it got to new levels when I got out of the military. I was on a couple different antidepressant medications. All the medications I was taking were just a temporary mask for my problems.

Ultimately, there were just too many side effects for me to continue taking them and I wanted to be off all medications, once and for all. The main side effect was feeling like a zombie with no drive, direction, or confidence. For the two years I was off the medications, I had these breakdowns whenever I was alone. I showed up and completed the things that needed to be done, but did this not being the best version of myself. It was not the version that I wanted to be for my family and team. I was falling apart on the inside. I was at the end of my rope. I was not in the driver's seat of my life anymore, and that was scary. Sometimes Depression can represent a lack of expression.

As I was trying to find the root of the problem, one doctor diagnosed me with severe social anxiety disorder. Once again, I was offered several medications to "level me out." But I immediately rejected them. I was not interested in going the medication route again.

Throughout the last several years of healing and post-traumatic growth, I have changed my relationship and how I frame and view depression. Some days are harder than others and I do get sad and cry and have emotions, but I allow myself and give myself permission to feel them and ride the waves of feelings and emotions.

Pattern interrupts are a super positive tool for me. I spend a lot of time with my dogs and outside in nature daily. Camping is another amazing pattern interrupt. Other pattern interrupts I keep in my back pocket are sound healing and obviously plant medicine journeys, both individual and group.

I find if I can fit in some combination of the following on a weekly basis, it really supports my mental health:

- Being in and around the water
- Striking/kickboxing
- Strength and conditioning
- Jiu jitsu

All these things are like therapy for me. They are critical for me being able to show up the best that I can for my family, companies, and team.

I had held in all my emotions and feelings before because I didn't know how to express or regulate and communicate my emotions to myself or others. I also didn't give myself permission to feel the feelings because I looked at myself as weak for being depressed and crying all the time. Before I was closed off and held everything in. Now, I communicate how I feel, which has required new levels of vulnerability and trust.

Mutually Symbiotic Relationships

There are all these different types of partnerships that exist within the plant and animal kingdoms that can be applied to human relationships in the highest form. Mutualistic symbiotic relationships are the best-case scenario. Think of strategic allies or alliances.

A mutualistic relationship occurs when two organisms of different species work together, each benefiting from the relationship, creating a win-win. An example in nature is the bee and the flower. The bee has freedom of movement while the flower has the supply. The bee transports the pollen from flower to flower, feeding the bee while allowing the plant to reproduce, resulting in a win-win situation.

It is part of the miracle of life to find the people who complement your weaknesses and counter your strengths. That's what makes great partnerships from my experience—powerful relationships and friendships bonded in finding ways to mutually support each other.

However, parasitic relationships are the worst case. A parasitic relationship in nature is when one organism (parasite) lives off another one. Parasites live on or in the body of the host. Sometimes we enable others by not creating boundaries from a toxic relationship. Healthy relationships are a two-way street—they are reciprocal in nature. The parasite and its host evolve together—the parasite adapts to its environment by living off the host in ways that harm and deteriorate the homeostasis and health of the host.

Over the years, we have experienced a multitude of challenges and obstacles dealing with different personalities in business environments who created different relational dynamics. And these parasitic relationships can become part of our comfort zone. It's important to continue to adapt and assess what's not working, and when necessary, find a support arm to assist you in getting the parasites off your back, when trying to shake them off yourself doesn't seem to work.

Hosts also develop ways of getting rid of parasites or protecting themselves from them. Some hosts even build a symbiotic relationship with another organism that helps in getting rid of the parasites.

Humans are creatures trying to observe and survive the patterns. You can choose to look at life through whatever frame you want. You can look at it like a nightmare or a miracle. You get to choose. And you get to choose how you put your energy and thoughts into different things so as a whole we progress forward in a more productive and healthy way.

When you realize the things that do need to be eliminated, it's best to approach with compassion and grace whenever possible.

During training and deployments as a Marine Raider, we embraced a motto of "Gung-Ho," which was the motto that the World War II Marine Raiders lived by, and in a lot of ways so did we . It is critical for small special operations teams to create mutually symbiotic relationships with their teammates and support elements to include all our partner forces in whatever country we are in.

Self-actualization includes aligning with our highest self. Identifying areas of growth within how we engage with self and others is critical in unlocking our highest potential.

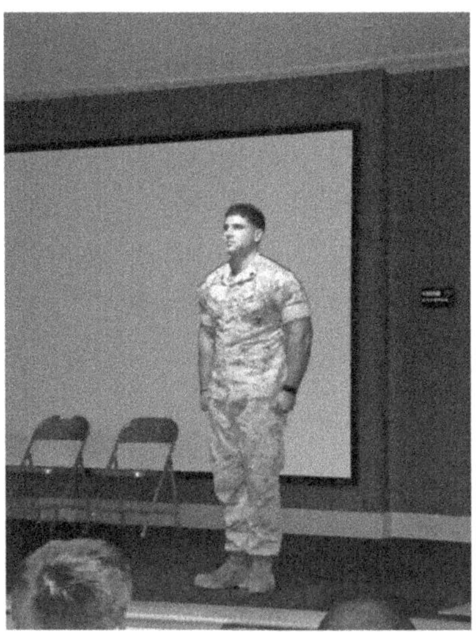

Receiving the Gung Ho Award—
Individual Training Course (2011)

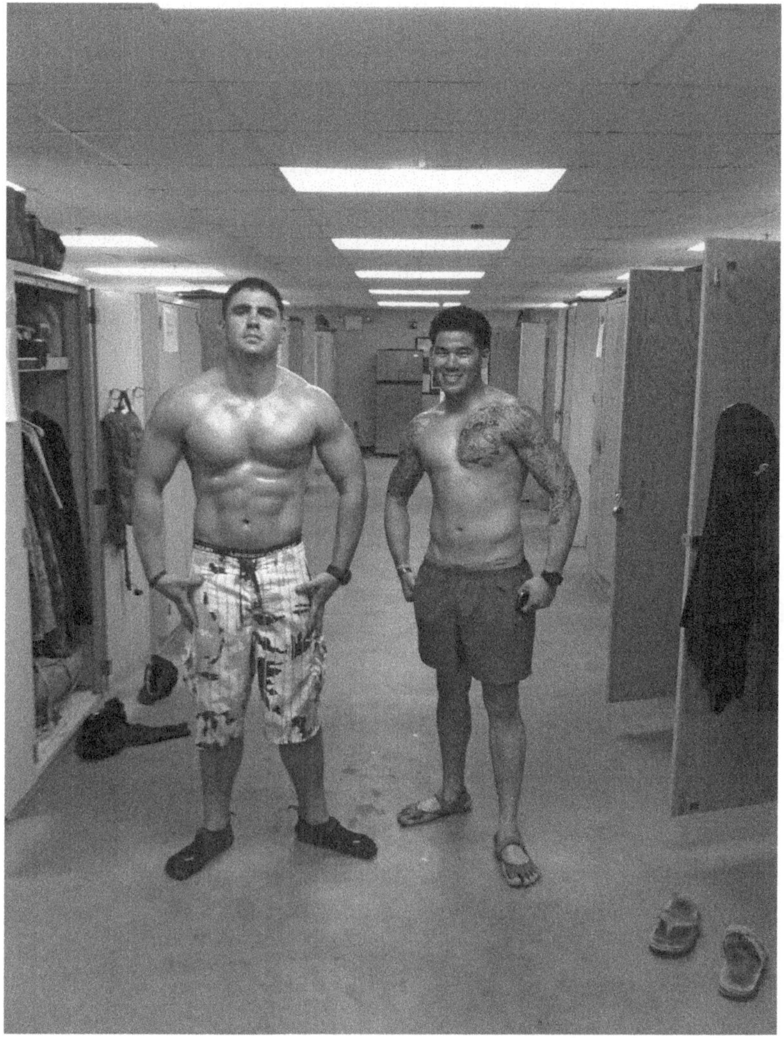

Prime with Don in the Raider Barracks During the Final Phase of Training (2011)

Dive Buddies

The stressful part of being a marine combatant diver is simply getting through dive school. After the course, all our dives were led by our own dive supervisors from our unit, who were always awesome to work with from my experience.

I got to be on the first official Marine Raider dive team, Marine Raider Team 8143. Our team motto, "Stay wet, stay hard," made us laugh and got us through many challenging situations with a positive outlook.

When we did night diving operations, you always had a buddy. You are essentially blacked out, underwater, with a nautical compass that glows in the dark that's attached to a navigation board/slate that you hold (called a *tactical board*). We had a piece of tape on it that we could write notes on. You had to strap into a carabiner to a buddy line for safety and to stay within close range of your buddy to carry out the dive and ensure you didn't get separated.

Another mantra we had when we strapped on the buddy line—as a reminder that you have to be alert and show up for you buddy—was "You are strapping into something bigger than yourself." In these dives, one guy would navigate, managing the depth of the dive and the other would be swimming.

We had a time and a target to hit. If we did not reach our target within the time allotted, we failed the dive. We were dropped off the coast of Florida. Some of the compasses were old and worn down. They sometimes locked up and got stuck during the dives and it took skill to keep the equipment working throughout the dives.

Sometimes when you are down there, you can start to doubt yourself, wondering *Am I on track?* We weren't allowed to break the surface on a dive, so if you thought you were lost, it was not as easy as coming up for air and seeing where you were in relation to the target. You had to stay calm and figure out the best direction based on all your assumptions of how long you had been diving in relation to your dive plan.

You go with a dive tank on, and a rebreather (oxygen circulates back into the tank so no bubbles come up). You are down there and breathing below water the whole time, using a Draeger (a re-breather dive tank that military use in stealth mode so there are no bubbles on the surface), kicking and finning as hard as you can, all while staying on track as best as possible. To keep the flow and stay on pace so that you hit the target on time, you do not want to be going up and down, changing depths frequently. It is up to your buddy to control the depth and make sure you stay as close to the planned depth as possible.

You plan your whole dive based on your depth, and how long you plan to be down there.

Sometimes there's a current or something holding you back that you need to navigate. If you are the navigator, you are in first player mode. Everything matters. You are the one dictating the path and the direction and setting the azimuth (the numbers on a compass in degrees that set the direction).

Let's say you go first. Then you're done and begin evaluated, and once you're checked off, how are you going to show up for your buddy? Are you going to go hang around and half ass just because you are off the hook? Or are you going to be present and a buddy and show up and support them? That was the other part of it: being a team player and working together or being Gung Ho. In fact, the surest way to get kicked out of Raider training was to be all about yourself and not work well with others. You don't always going to agree with every decision made, but that doesn't mean you sabotage the leadership and you don't put your best effort out to support the team. These were all simple, but valuable lessons that translate into working in any team environment: military, business, sports, and so on. These principles always apply.

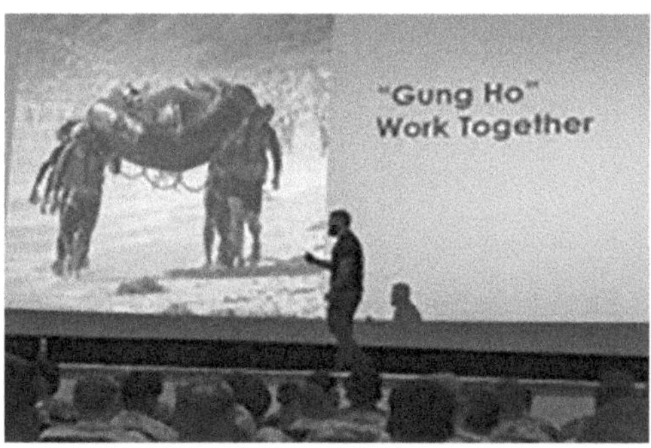

Prime Speaking to the Marines at Camp Pendleton (2024)

CHAPTER 11

Relationships and Integration

For anyone struggling with depressive or suicidal thoughts, in the darkest moments, it's so important to know that even in the final round of the fight, even in the last seconds of the fight, you can still win. Your life is not over.

You Can Still Win in the Final Round of the Fight

Don't isolate yourself.

Don't give up on yourself.

Don't give up the fight.

Push the fight.

In the military and in special ops, missions are often planned off a worst-case scenario, which creates the opportunity to build contingency plans, mitigate, and navigate whatever the enemy might do, based on their capabilities and the most probable courses of action.

The worst-case scenario for veterans is an increasing number of suicides year after year, and we are all deeply saddened and affected by every life lost to suicide. There is one suicide death almost every 10 minutes in the United States across the total population. In the world, there is one suicide every 40 seconds. Most are males.

Within the veteran community, I've heard countless stories of men who operated at the highest levels of the military, who deployed

145

around the world, carrying out some of the most dangerous missions imaginable. But the worst danger often doesn't come until they transition. For many, the risk of suicide in quiet suburban neighborhoods was greater than anything they faced in the most war-torn of environments. That truth hit me hard.

It was my experience, too. That's why, after hearing story after story of suicide, I knew I couldn't stay silent. No matter how uncomfortable it is to share my own story, staying quiet is no longer an option.

In business school after getting out of the military, I sat in class asking myself, *Is this really what life is going to be all about? Are most days in my future going to involve me being indoors under bright, artificial lights?* Sitting in classes trying to focus on something "important" like statistics was a challenge for me mentally and physically. I had sharp pains in my back every time I moved. I was also inundated with thoughts from different traumatic events. Even with all the medications I was on, I was in pure misery.

I don't think there was ever a split second while I was in Afghanistan that I would have ever recognized any kind of depression or thought about killing myself. I was in pure survival mode and had a lot of coping mechanisms to deal with the stress. We got attacked every day. It wasn't until I got home and got out that I started to realize how difficult transitioning was; it made overseas missions seem simple. Everything seemed so seamless in the military . . . it was only once we got back was when I was really in the most dangerous situation of all.

I put myself into a lot of dangerous situations during my transition. Hitting rock bottom after getting out of the military, I constantly put myself into situations and environments that were dangerous.

Being in the most dangerous situations on deployment was almost like I had a security blanket. Everyone on my team was extremely effective and capable, especially some of the senior guys. Even being a new guy, I was in a safe place because they had all the experience and were great leaders to have. They gave the team more confidence to navigate the adversity that we were up against.

I never contemplated suicide while on active duty. I was sad about certain things, but I did not experience depression. It wasn't until I got home that I started having those problems. Even more so when I got out of the military.

I first started getting depressed when I got put on the medical review board. I was off duty and away from my team. Sometimes I went to medical appointments three to four times a day. Sometimes at those appointments I had to do things until I get extremely nauseous. It felt as if I had no meaning. I was just going to medical appointments and all my meaning was gone. And that's how transition started to get kind of dicey at this point. I had all this trauma but no meaning. Now I was out in the world after all these crazy experiences.

Transitioning from anything in which you have an identity or a purpose that makes you a contributing member of society, when that gets taken from you, it needs to be acknowledged. You can know that it's coming, and you will have to redefine what your meaning is and realign with that new thing. And that may not happen overnight.

Any way you can, open your mind and get outside the box. Go to seminars and courses; go on vacation. A change in scenery can help unlock new perspectives. Give yourself permission to allow a new frequency and place of possibility than what would be there when immediately getting out.

Business on Life Support

Going into 2020. We had crazy momentum and growth in Deep End Fitness and Underwater Torpedo League. We had investors lined up, so much media, public relations, and partnerships—everything was taking off for us. *The Today Show* came out for a weekend at the pool to tell our story. The story never aired because when COVID-19 hit, all momentum *stopped*. We halted everything, like the rest of the world. That put us on life support.

We did everything that we could to continue training and find any opportunity to do what we do. We did ocean training or trained in private pools. We focused on working with instructors and elite athletes who had competitions or other high-level stuff still going on. But this put us in a very, very challenging spot. Toward the end of 2020 we decided to jump-start everything and get momentum going again.

Survival Versus Meaning

Sometimes things are truly out of your control, and that's a scary time. I gained a lot of clarity through this time of great uncertainty, and it made me think a lot about and investigate survival and meaning.

John Danaher, arguably the best jiu jitsu coach in the world, talks about how humans are the most adaptable creatures on earth, able to adjust to nearly anything. We have broken through from learning while in survival mode.

We're not in survival mode like we were thousands of years ago. But we're in a different kind of survival stage now. What's crazy is that in earlier stages of humanity, there wasn't suicide like there is today, because everyone was focusing on survival. Just like soldiers actively in war are not thinking about killing themselves, it's usually not until later when processing their experiences do they reach the end of their rope.

In today's culture, we're not in survival mode with all the Uber Eats, Urgent Care, air conditioning, Zoom meetings, and other technologies. Everything is a one click, buy, or swipe away. Survival looks different. There's no hunting and gathering, and social interactions have been diminished as we struggle to balance technological advancements with how we relate to each other as fellow humans and the environment around us.

With the luxuries and conveniences of today, survival is now about meaning and connection. It's about designing more healthy and productive ways of finding purpose and meaning. When people get off track and lose all sense of meaning, they are most susceptible to suicide.

I find the most meaning when I am helping others unlock potential and reach goals. It's when I put too much focus on myself that I start to get out of alignment. But when I am outwardly focused on whom I can help, it creates the best flow for me in all areas of life. Of course, I still need to take care of myself and keep my own oxygen mask on. However, I'm in a better space and take better care of myself when I am in an outward-focused place in life.

A simple exercise I use to take me from inward focused to outward focused immediately is to ask myself, *Who is one person I can make a difference to right now?* Because there is always somebody in life that you can reach out to and support or cheer up. When you focus out and support others, and you take action to help make a positive impact in their life, you will quickly shift your own state.

If finding meaning is still a challenge, seeking feedback from key people is a strategic tool that we always have in our tool belt to help. This is important so that we can see how others perceive us and how we show up for them in comparison to how we think we show up. We get to see our blind spots and gaps when we get authentic feedback from people who care about us. Ask trusted people in your life.

Whatever you find to be the most meaningful thing to you—your life, your mind, your consciousness, your day, your week—notice it and align all these things to what your meaning is.

Part of my soul mission is to create a positive shift in humanity. To coach the best in the world as they do what they do. To make my family proud. These goals ground me in purpose, which keeps me focused and aligned day-to-day as I approach certain obstacles. I have a strong why that can carry me through and reshape challenges into opportunities. When I feel off track or out of alignment I go back to my why or purpose.

Going back to the most meaningful things keeps me in a positive flow. This is what I think of as daily and weekly maintenance— the integration work—and continuing to heal and not getting complacent or comfortable thinking I have already done the work. My inner work will always continue and is likely never going to be complete.

What are we doing in our society? What direction are we moving? As technology advances, it seems that the attention span of humanity continues to decrease. The more we immerse ourselves with technology, you can argue that we get farther away from nature and the source. It's disruptive to our human needs, causing depression and keeping humans out of alignment with any type of meaning in life.

If technology disrupts our human needs and connection with each other and the natural world, what can we do to counteract this to find balance in our lives in between the physical and the unseen spiritual worlds?

Having a strong why and purpose is like having a shield. My meaning is my family. For my grandparents, parents, wife, kids, or my extended family, I will do anything. If the why for doing anything is about me, I have noticed that I will not go as far or stretch myself as far as I will if it's not outwardly focused on someone else.

Purpose and meaning keep me grounded and in alignment with my highest self.

Calm Seas Never Make Strong Sailors

I've always related to the eagle as a spirit animal. It can fly high or fly low and gains different perspectives going through hardship. I try to think with the perspective of an eagle when I look at moving through rough seas.

From my own perspective, some moments of life and business have been uncomfortable. I have felt hopeless many times. Those rough seas I can now translate to add value to other people's lives. And I would not have been able to this if I had not been through those experiences. It enables me to work with athletes preparing to fight or defend world championships, clients who have huge challenges or opportunities on the line. I can translate frameworks from any of the pattern recognition that I have from any of those experiences.

Those became some of the most valuable lessons I have learned personally that give me confidence to support others.

Working with some of these individuals is inspiring. One of my favorite clients is the CEO of an elite sports agency/management firm that has worked with and represented some of the top Ultimate Fighting Championship fighters in the world. There are things that he deals with that are crazy. He has big ups and sometimes it seems like he is in rough seas. But that's what makes him a strong sailor. This experience has made him the best in the world at what he does. He is a champion in my eyes.

With whatever season of life, you are going through, it can feel like you are in rough seas. Reframing that as quickly as you can helps you navigate it differently. Sometimes it gets frustrating with obstacles and rough seas. But at the end of the day, everyone wants to be the sailor who adds value and contributes to humanity.

Life happens. Things can go from 0 to 100 fast. Everything can be smooth sailing and suddenly there is a health problem. A car accident takes a loved one. In combat things can turn on a moment's notice. In the ocean, a nice day can abruptly end with a drowning or someone getting smashed against the pier. The seas can go from calm to rough in an instant. What can you do when the seas get rough? You can't always prepare for these moments, but these actions can help:

1. Gather your support circle: mentors, friends, family.
2. Train your body and your mind to deal with rough seas.
3. Identify processes and frameworks for problem-solving that work for you. A strengths, weaknesses, opportunities, threats (SWOT) analysis works for me, as do OSMEAC (a military planning tool that stands for orientation, situation, mission, execution, administration/logistics, command/signal) or a primary, alternate, contingency, emergency (PACE) plan.

I provide more details on my website about the SWOT, OSMEAC, and PACE frameworks.

When rough seas hit, you want to have these things built out. You want to be trained and have a prepared mind. You want to have tools and processes in your tool belt. You don't want to figure this out as the seas go from calm to rough. You want to have done this training so you don't get seasick anymore. You can do a full shift and can last in a positive mindset. You can do two shifts if you need to. You've conditioned your mind and you are in flow. You have found calm in the storm.

It's like the backwards law. Sometimes the more we try to force an outcome or achievement, the more it slips away. The law suggests that letting go of outcomes and accepting the flow of life is what unlocks the most results and achievement. Sometimes our mind wants to have a bright sunny day with the calm sea and beautiful sunset. But how can we train our minds so that we can be at that same level of peace when we hit the rough seas, like in hell week in the military, or whatever other scenario that we might have to face?

Once Upon a Time in Tijuana

I went for a stem cell treatment once and it was my first time in Tijuana (TJ). I drove my 4Runner there with Don Tran and our good friend Ryan Spadafore, thinking it would be easy to navigate using Google Maps. We stayed at an Airbnb on Tijuana Beach near the hospital. On the second night we were there, we were invited to a dinner with a bunch of other athletes.

Don decided to stay at the Airbnb to finish some work, but Ryan and I drove to the dinner spot, which happened to be close to the entry point to go back to the United States.

Heading back to the Airbnb after dinner, we took a wrong turn and accidentally went back toward the border and ended up in the line to cross back into California. It would have taken five or six hours to get across and then cross back into Mexico to get back to our Airbnb.

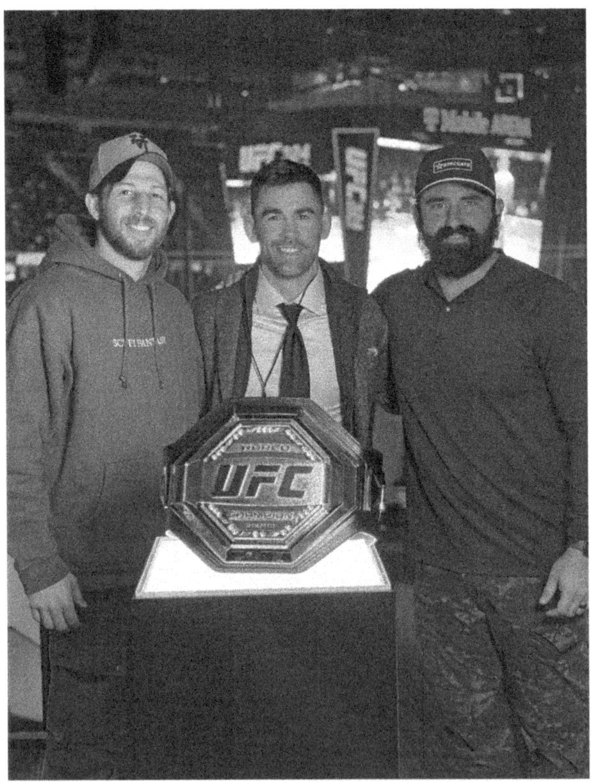

Prime with Dom Cruz and Ryan Spadafore (2026) at
Dom's UFC Hall of Fame Induction

I could not see myself sitting in that line for six hours to then driving back. One of my pet peeves is wasted or inefficient movements, so when we got over this hill and saw that we're about to get funneled into a line of thousands of cars, I felt panic kicking in. At the same time, I immediately turned right, and there was a group of merchants along the far side of the road who were selling gum and souvenirs to cars leaving Mexico.

I asked a group of them in broken Spanish, "Is there any way to get back to Tijuana Beach, to la Playa?" They immediately said yes that it was possible, but we would need to go really slow, stay to the right side of the road, and as soon as we see the turn, we have to turn right and drive fast.

I started driving toward the interstate driving into oncoming traffic while blinking my hazard lights on and flashing everyone, keeping a close eye for the turn the merchants told us about. We didn't see the turn, and we were getting increasingly anxious. We had gone so far that we had to keep going. But that was one of the craziest experiences. Thankfully we remained calm and didn't hit any cars or get caught by a policia. We finally made it to the turn and made it back to the Airbnb. We filled Don in on what happened, laughing as we told the story.

Keeping with the mindset of making it happen and finding a way, laughter has always been a secret power for me to deal with pain and stress. In one of my most chaotic moments—the insider attack—we laughed at anything and everything that we could. Sure, we were partly concussed. But trying to laugh during some of the most chaotic moments is one way to cope. This reminds me of one of my favorite sayings, "Do not forget to sing in the lifeboats."

Coping

You're in rough seas or are going back and forth between calm and rough seas. Or you might be in calm seas but start getting nightmares about the rough seas. Sometimes there is stress you need to cope with.

So how do we cope? Again, we approach versus avoid. In these moments, it is beneficial to ask whether we are we actively approaching them, communicating about them, and working to break through them.

Otherwise, the next step is masking them, which can lead to many unhealthy choices. So now, based on how we're coping, we find ways to mask and shove the issues aside, which will emerge in other ways that tend to be destructive to self or others.

Sometimes you have people in your life who are toxic. It doesn't mean that you have to block them. But make sure to put boundaries on them for your own sanity and well-being. Just make sure you are not avoiding the message or figuring out why this person is toxic. What's the download for that? How is any resistance or relationship that's not working or toxic? How can you find a mirror in this situation or a person who can be useful for you in your life? How can you learn from this?

Circle of Trust

I've learned it's always important to have a 360° security system in place. You should have it in all directions around you, especially if in a contested combat zone. You don't want any vulnerabilities from any angle around your position. It's important to also build a 360° security in your life with your relationships before you transition out of the military. Family or other support systems are critical; you can think of this as your perimeter. These commitments can keep you grounded and secure from taking a dangerous path and staying on the right path and not veering off. Think of this as your perimeter in life or your safety net.

Vision Board and Manifestation

Creating vision boards is a simple yet powerful way to begin to identify and manifest your truest desires and help you avoid traps that are not in alignment with your truest purpose Write down your goals and visions until it becomes ingrained in your subconscious mind. I also recommend creating an online vision board to bring your vision to life and begin to paint your own reality.

Avoid Golden Handcuffs

The keynote speaker at a conference I attended talked about the concept of golden handcuffs. It's stuck with me ever since. The speaker was asked about when he decided to leave his job and start his own company. He responded that when he was *really* ready to leave a job, the company tried to give him golden handcuffs to keep him working there longer. And eventually he could see through that, which enabled him to finally make the move he wanted.

This hit home for me. It's hard to create a positive shift in your mental health if you are miserable in your work environment or in a relationship, friendship, or whatever. Miserable dynamics like these are all examples of golden handcuffs. The golden handcuff could be a job or any other thing that keeps you tied to something for the security of a certain title, salary, or other element of social or ego-based gain.

The biggest issue that I help people getting out of the military with is deciding which job to take. Don't compromise—go after what you know will give your purpose and meaning. Don't just jump into a box and check it. Like, "I only need a job to make me x/year." It's a horrible way to find your purpose.

Anxiety and Relief

When I went to military school, I became an insomniac, going for days without sleeping, and not sleeping a lot when I did. From 17 to 19 I had real patterns of insomnia. I went to the doctor, and they gave me Xanax bars. I lived on the border of Mexico and would go to the pharmacia in Mexico and get these bars.

I would take Xanax to mask anxiety and avoid everything that caused me stress. Even simple situations like going to the movies or out to a restaurant. There is no prize at the end of that rainbow. I see it as a self-licking ice cream cone. Sure, it brings immediate reward because it masks everything, but you are actually moving backwards in life. Instead of approaching, you are avoiding. I was avoiding life.

As I've mentioned, I started masking with alcohol at school for my master of business administration program. When you are usually a high performer, and people can see you're not being yourself and are way off the normal baseline of how you usually show up, it should create some red flags with the people who care about you.

Each time I had serious side effects or pain, the doctors tried to prescribe me yet another medication. I wanted to be aware of my anxiety as much as possible so I could manage it.

If you are looking to manage anxiety, ask yourself, *What is the number one activity that I can do daily that relieves it?*

There are several things that work for me. For one, when I do underwater training, I am completely relaxed for the rest of the day. I come out with way less anxiety and more joy as I head into the rest of my day. As a water enthusiast, I love being in the water, so I find a way to make this part of my life on a regular basis. It also relieves my anxiety.

In recent years, I like to do jiu jitsu in the morning a couple times a week as an outlet to clear my emotional state and evolve as a person. This sets up my day for total success on the mental front. I always leave the workout emotionally, physically, psychologically, and spiritually better.

Another thing I do is regularly check in on my mindset. How clear is my mental operating system? I ask myself, *How much digital detox have I done lately? Do I need more? Am I taking in too much information? Do I need an information diet?*

If I notice the TV is always on, or the radio never stops, or I feel uncomfortable without constant background noise, that's usually a sign I need to unplug. I look at my own consciousness and ask, is there too much clutter? What can I take away—or what can I add—that would help create more clarity and flow in my life?

Since getting out of the military I have gone into deep exploration on what practices unlock the most clarity and support my mental focus throughout the day. What practices can you do daily or weekly to defrag your mind? Another activity for me is mediation. Most days I meditate at least once, if not twice or more. Rise and meditate in the morning and start with a clear operating system, proactively approaching the day. Do something so you're not waking up in reaction mode. Mediate first thing in the morning and right after work so you sandwich it. Take a mental snapshot of your awareness and how clear it is. Then you can make a list of anything that gives you anxiety in your life. Then ask what is one action that you can take for each one of those items that brings you anxiety.

All these things can be done in moderation or in small steps, and sometimes you can use them in more advanced ways as you work them into your life in a strategic way to help address anxiety.

One way to pattern interrupt is to cut everything out with sensory deprivation. Like a float tank, something I use when I need a reset.

It's like locking yourself into a little cell where there is no sensory stimulation, which is helpful because sometimes, when you are trying to look out, you actually need to look inside.

For some, getting into a sensory deprivation tank may take some serious working up to. For an athlete, it may need to be something more shocking or extreme. I know of an athlete who spends three to five days alone in a completely dark room before going into a fight camp. He uses this practice to strip everything down and find his true sense of self and get a true pattern interruption. So, for three-plus days, he goes with no light or sense of time whatsoever. You only know what time it is when you open the door and it's done.

I've had people I work with who have claustrophobia being a float tank. I think this is a good example of an opportunity to step into your power. Find a way to create a process in your mind to face the fear and work through the challenge. Your anxiety will go down, and you will have more confidence.

And, as I've discussed elsewhere, I've found that my strongest interrupt was plant medicine. If you go down that path, do your research and set intentions. The pattern interrupt is the journey. But there is still integration after that.

Dealing with Resistance

Everyone I know deals with anxiety to some extent, which can stem from all kinds of different fears and our relationship to that fear. The best thing to do is to face that fear, such as my fear of heights—which came from my fall as a child. I did civilian skydiving because I wanted to approach that fear. Every time I stepped out of the plane, that fear and anxiety was conquered a little bit more. Sometimes it's a matter of running toward the gunfire, right into the thing that gives resistance.

It is important to ask yourself, *Where is my resistance coming from?* Sometimes it's stuff we make up in our mind. And we build up these situations in our heads. We create illusions and give way too much power to something that simply is not a real threat to us. A lot of our emotions are held in our stories. What stories have you told yourself that are holding you back?

Sometimes we live in negative stories in our minds, but when we actually break them down on paper and face them in real life, they lose power. The more we can connect to the awareness part of our consciousness, we start to see how our mind play tricks on us. Our mind is always looking to find reasons for things. There are times I feel in resistance with my own mind, because my mind is simply being a survival mechanism and wanting to keep me safe or assign meaning to everything in my life.

Your ego is always looking for ways to be right. Knowing how your mind works and being aware of it is foundational. You start to see where the traps come in and how your mind plays tricks on you. You also start to notice what stories are holding you back and creating anxiety.

A good practice is to list stories you tell yourself about your anxieties. Then, list powerful attributes about yourself. Next, cancel out the anxieties with the powerful attributes you know about yourself. Cancel out the bullshit and disprove your anxieties by owning your strengths. It can be helpful to ask other people who know you well to list these powerful attributes and help disprove the anxieties that are holding you back.

When I first approached by anxieties, I realized it's more simple than I thought it would be. That's because in the mind it can feel unsolvable, but when you put it on paper and start to identify it, you can see what the real gap is between where you are and what you want or need to be. It becomes more clear to see the action steps and form a plan, which helps eliminate anxiety.

For example, *If I sign up for (fill in the blank), it will be a step toward self-mastery*. Write down the goal. Then identify the gap or the thing you feel is holding you back or is in the way. Maybe it's a commitment of your time, energy, and/or money. Once you know the gap, ask somebody to be your accountability partner. Then put yourself into the gap and work every day to get closer to your goal.

Another thing that is simple, but not easy, is cleaning up your thought garden. When I need to do this, I look at all the little things I tell myself that I will do. Sometimes I don't do them, and when that happens, I lose trust in myself, and it creates weeds in the thought garden. This is when my operating system starts to degrade and I have to build confidence again to remove the doubt and clean the garden.

Keeping your word to yourself is so important. So, if I say I'm going to wake up and run, I build trust and faith in myself when I wake up and go for that run. Keeping your word to yourself is key to helping you stay aligned with your strategic goals and purpose. It's the start of a ripple effect. I love the book *The Four Agreements: A Practical Guide to Personal Freedom* by Don Miguel Ruiz (Tarcher, 1997) for a deeper dive on the power of keeping your word to yourself.

Once you are aware and intentional, then pattern interrupt can be reinforced. A military example would be stop, listen, look, smell. We used this practice to become fully present and aware of our environment. For example, we would walk with a 150-pound backpack and a machine gun through a minefield in Afghanistan at night to get to an enemy village. When approaching the village we would take a knee; stop, look, listen, and smell to get our bearings; and become fully engaged with the environment.

It's normal to have anxiety about the future. When I try to control the future, it creates a lot of anxiety for me. A lot of this is self-induced, removing me from flow.

Breath work tools can be powerful in these moments. On my website I list several that can help break the pattern and shift your focus and mindset, including one called *jailbreaking your mind*.

High Speed, Low Drag

Clutter can be a huge source of drag. I've found it important to declutter my mind and environment as much as possible. Taking time to declutter any area of life (office, car, garage, etc.) can improve your quality of life and help you release drag. What you do in one area, you do in all.

If my car is a mess, if my garage is not organized, it causes me mental clutter and slows me down. Less is more for me. The same goes for technology and notifications. All my technology is set up with specific settings, so I don't constantly have noises going on and distractions popping up. I often have my phone on silent and have it go straight to voicemail because there's a big switching cost when I need to focus. I have a process for urgent things too. But, when possible, I eliminate distractions, so I have a clear stream of consciousness, and my mind is like a blank canvas.

For me, especially with traumatic brain injury, having things as simple as possible supports me and how I perform in my daily activities and duties at work and at home. I was told by doctors that I would struggle just to find my keys for the rest of my life. That is far from the case, but the practice of keeping things simple is good for anyone and everyone. Simple habits and rituals help me with this. For instance, I like to declutter on Sundays because it sets up my week for success. I keep my clothing options simple by having limited options on what to wear. I mostly wear the same thing day-to-day, almost like my own uniform, which makes for less of a cognitive load to carry.

I relate how my mind works to a computer or smartphone operating system. Humans are not born with a physical operating manual, but I believe it's inside of each of us and it's up to us to unlock it. All the answers are inside. We live in a world that moves so fast it can be hard to see it and access it. However, you can find that access point with intentional practices, such as meditation, prayer, stillness, time in nature, or isolation.

Controlling how you manage your cognitive/mental bandwidth is also important. How can you set different boundaries so you have more bandwidth? Anxiety is a big source of drag. Can you identify what is creating self-induced anxiety or what your external sources of anxiety are? What social media creates stress and anxiety. What mental drag can you eliminate to enhance your operating system? This exercise is important because it increases cognitive bandwidth and horsepower while supporting mental health and overall well-being. If the news or politics bother me, I go on a low-info diet. Divisive media and politics can drain your spirit and drag you down. Why spend your energy fighting battles that don't serve your purpose? Instead, focus on meaningful connections and purpose-driven actions that uplift you and those around you.

To revisit the thought garden. Like a jail-broken mind, it doesn't grow weeds if abundant plants are filling up the garden. The weeds don't matter, they just become obsolete.

Avoiding Entropy

Lack of order or predictability can take gradual decline into complete disorder. It's important, because it goes back to the saying, "How you do one thing is how you do everything." If my outer world is cluttered it starts to take over into the inner world and mental clutter. This is why I am constantly organizing and decluttering my spaces and simultaneously my mind. Meditation and silence help to quiet the mind.

It's the little things being out of order that can create disorder in life. To me, these small things matter and they add up quickly.

Reset is a process. Sometimes it requires making a big mess to take everything out and create complete order. When this happens, clean the room and put everything back in.

Other times, little things create disorder in life, like your car just needs to be vacuumed. Our mind can make these little things more than they are because they are seeking survival. The mind can jump to predicting things that do not match up with reality.

Love over Fear

My favorite author and speaker Wayne Dyer said, "Fear knocked at the door. Love answered. No-one was there."

The two root emotions that we all have are love and fear. It's a superpower to have the awareness and ability to understand what emotions drive our actions and know if we are coming from a place of love or fear. I've noticed that when I focus on the wrong things, it's critical to shift out of that mindset. Sometimes my ego starts to feel like it's playing tricks on me. I try to notice it the best I can and surrender it and let it go. I try to remember that I am not my ego; I am working more into being the observer. I notice that my mind frames things in survival mode a lot. I can manage the survival part of the mind a lot more than the ego part. I find it extremely helpful to shift my focus onto others I care about, focusing on love instead of fear.

This requires noticing what emotion is coming from the ego and letting it go. Every now and then something happens or some type of relationship obstacle creates this emotional baggage or stress, which can be a trap. Sometimes you'll start to focus on yourself instead of what the other person did, and that's a fool's errand.

Once you notice that you're focused on something not working for you, practice the ability to shift and refocus on yourself. Imagine looking at a target through a scope of a rifle. How can you shift and refocus your attention and energy off yourself and onto somebody you care about?

CHAPTER 12

Ripple Effects of Positive Change

In Seth Godin's book *The Dip: A Little Book That Teaches You When to Quit (and When to Stick)* (Portfolio, 2007), he talks about how everything worth getting good at has a dip in the middle of that progress. The dip is when things get tough and you stop making easy progress. This is when your growth can slow to a crawl and when you are most likely to give up on your goals.

Plan for the Dip

One benefit of being under a lot of pressure is that after a while it starts to sharpen you. Sometimes pressure can knock you down and break you down, but you can work through that dip. The super pressure of a dip helped unlock things I never thought possible for myself: an opportunity to turn some very difficult times into something beautiful.

I remember the feeling of getting through the dip and completing certain courses within the marine special operations training pipeline. Completing hell week, jump school, dive school (which I had failed before), Marine Raider selection, and individual training course, and some survival, evasion, resistance, and escape schools.

During these courses I had multiple ego deaths, a personal drowning scare, multiple injuries that really made me question myself, and moments where I was on the edge of failing or dropping out. But I just continued to show up and make it through the dip.

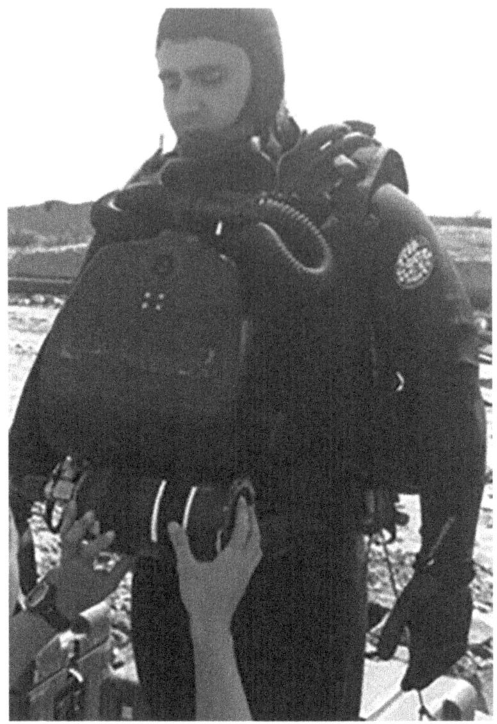

Combatant Dive Training, Camp Pendleton, California (2014)

Even a Broken Clock Is Right Twice a Day

I continue to face challenges and obstacles, even when writing this book, and sometimes they almost feel impossible. My favorite thing to remember when things are tough, or when it's hard to tell if the right decisions are being made, is that even a broken clock is right twice a day. Even if you are a "broken clock" as a person, sometimes you're going to get it right.

If you find yourself in a high-stress situation or dealing with anxiety about a task that feels impossible (because you are not taking action), it can be helpful to break it down into smaller, more manageable goals or action steps.

It is hard sometimes to see people's true colors and to see who is who in the zoo, especially when everything is smooth sailing. You really find out who your people are when you face challenges or are compromised in some way. Injuries bring vulnerability. Real friends are like night vision or flashlights in the darkness.

Every time we get high visibility from our work with different athletes or teams we are training at Deep End Fitness (DEF), I usually get some feedback along the lines of "Oh wow, Prime, *now* you're doing it!" But the reality is, we've been at this for a while now, and the results are just starting to be seen on a larger scale. Maybe we, as a team and organization, are close to passing the dip.

What is possible? We never know what's possible because tomorrow hasn't happened or played out yet. I don't know what those things will be. But in the meantime, to get through the dip, it's important to pay attention to what we are tuning into.

We Don't Know What We Don't Know

The Johari window is a technique to develop more self-awareness, designed to help people better understand their relationship with themselves and others. This can also be used to compare what you consider to be your own strengths and weaknesses to others' perceptions of them. I share a demonstration of this in the Resources.

If somebody is not in a state of awareness to receive the information you are trying to give them, it's going to be hard to deliver that message. In our modern society, there seems to be so much messaging and chaotic noise in every direction that you look. Propaganda about election candidates, wars, rap beefs, and constant information operations put out through the media and popular culture are all energy sucks that will rob your spirit if you allow it to. Seek out people who are rising above the noise and breaking out of the mold.

When I use the word *matrix*, I am referring to the media and culture in the present day. Media outlets of all kinds create influence and control over a population, whether good or bad, such as if you are watching the news and it's always reporting a tragedy for us to get sucked into and rob our spirits. There is usually a false projection of some type: disease, war, famine, fires, and so on. Whenever I talk to anyone back home from Texas, they ask if I am okay because they see all the news about different things in my area in California. I have to explain to them that it's not real. I see this all as a distraction from connecting with your higher self and doing what you are supposed to do in life. In the military we would label these activities information ops.

Mental Focus

Mental acuity means to be mentally sharp in all energy and operations relating to the process of thinking—everything from information processing to memory, attention, situational awareness, and judgment. Keeping your mental sword sharp requires effort because cognitive abilities can decline with age or after a brain injury.

Lack of mental acuity creates a dull sword and can become a health detriment. It can mean you forget important things and lose the ability to perform tasks, losing cognitive bandwidth and function.

Increasing your mental acuity doesn't have to be complicated. Sometimes, it's a matter of eliminating choices or simplifying things. Focus on small victories and creating little wins every day to create flow.

Just as important are the things we should incorporate, there are also many things that can drain our mental acuity. Too much artificial light or screen time drain us. I include a list of recommendations for optimal brain health and mental acuity in the Resources section.

Living with Authority

At a certain point, we all have to take charge of our own life. When you experience hardships and integrate and work through something really challenging, it can bring new levels of knowledge, experience, and authority in that area. If you are in transition from an institution like the military, it can be very challenging to move and act in the civilian world with confidence.

With the experiences I have had and by studying others, I've stepped into a new level of authority, which is something I do not take lightly. I consider it a responsibility to provide resources to others who are navigating those same waters that I did.

Beginning is often the *most* challenging part to start addressing and facing traumas. To heal the trauma, we must address it. Sometimes a re-injury can cause us to reexperience it, which can be painful. However, if we commit to work through it, *freedom* is waiting for us on the other side of the painful emotion.

I have been much better about framing anything and everything that happens in a positive light. When the Afghan war ended, and the way that America pulled out in August 2021, I saw it cause a lot of breakdowns in my community. I cared deeply for the Afghan people, as did a lot of our military who lived and fought side by side with them. It was hurtful to see how it all unfolded. I do my best to focus on the honor, service, and sacrifice of so many, and the amazing acts that I witnessed when I was there instead of going down the rabbit hole of "why this?" and "why that?", which can lead to downward spiral and mental health crash.

In my experience, it feels like the survival part of my mind is always working to assign meaning to every little thing. Something is usually classified as either good or bad, and someone is right or wrong (ego). If you can look at life from the viewpoint of an observer, everything that happens in life is neutral. It is only our reaction to and emotion about each event that takes it out of neutrality.

Traumas Can Be Teachers

We're all here as humans and we are all here figuring it out. We were not born with an operating manual or guidebook on how to live our lives in the most optimal way and work through our relationship with ourself and with others. It's okay to have allowance and grace for yourself and others in the process. There is a lot of freedom and other gifts on the other side of forgiveness. Yes, you can have forgiveness and grace for others who have wronged you. It doesn't mean you ever have to see them again, but you can forgive them. The forgiveness process is cathartic for *you* to let go of any cancer or poison that you carry from any resentment against another person. Don't poison yourself with resentment and expect the other person will suffer. That is the opposite of how it works.

Developing positive coping skills to deal with traumas is critical to your overall well-being and livelihood. Even in my own healing, and after I had what I call my rebirth, I came back, and wow, I'm in my new life. But that's not the end of it, when working with my integration coach, Dr. Michelle, she started asking about my childhood traumas again, and that created a lot of pain. At first it felt like reinjury, experiencing the pain and trauma from the past. And my advice for when this thing happens is to allow yourself to *be open* and take all the feedback and every last bit of learning that can come from it. If I am not open, I close myself off and bury my problems, which I know very well *is not the answer*. The other thing that worked for me was accountability with her, my other coaches, and people I am close with.

I have an amazing respect and trust for all my coaches. As I began my healing journey, I learned that I had a lot of traumas that I had not addressed. When I started working with Dr. Michelle, we began pulling a lot of this information out. If I didn't have that respect and trust, I would not be able to go deep and access all the emotions. Another huge gift of having coaches is the accountability and support that a strong coach provides. I have had a lot of sessions and opportunities to lean in and deal with past traumas, expose them, face them, and start to heal and learn from them.

I continue to share this kind of vulnerable information as I continue my mission to build resolve and resilience in others, destigmatizing asking for help when it's needed to save families and save lives.

Forgiveness

When it comes to finding forgiveness, whenever I personally struggle with dealing with someone, I try to remember an emotional intelligence training session that I attended. We were shown a picture of an iceberg. Only a small part is above the water. The largest part of an iceberg is underneath the water.

When you have an issue with another person, ask yourself or them about what they facing are or dealing with that is underneath the surface, hidden from what you can see. You will gain compassion and understanding that helps put the overall situation into perspective. I find this to be a deeper route to forgiveness.

Some people get lost in the fog or drunk at the party; I know I have been there. Another way of finding compassion is to frame and accept what somebody did in another light and recognize they likely did not have the awareness or tools to make better decisions. They were lost in the fog. This will help you not to become resentful. You may even appreciate them as a gift.

It has been challenging at times to process different things and reach a place of forgiveness. I am still bothered by some of the experiences I had as a kid. Through a lot of healing work and integration I have been able to *shift* my perspective on much of it.

A shift in perspective and reframe is what has guided me through the chaos. The events that happened shaped and molded me into the person I am today.

One positive development that happened after I went to my first healing ceremony was that I went back to my old house where I grew up and where I had experienced the peeping Tom.

It was amazing to see that the new owners had built a fence around the entire side of the house where my bedroom window was. Even though I had not lived in that house for nearly 30 years, it was a powerful visual and moment for me to see the fence there; I will never forget it. To know that there's no way that anyone there could ever watch a child or anyone through that window gave me peace and allowed part of me to heal. I share these things with the intent that it will open up an opportunity for others to heal and find peace.

I highly recommend to anyone who lives in a house, and especially anyone who has kids, to be mindful of your landscaping and window access to your kids' rooms. Don't create an opportunity where somebody can come up to the windows. Ideally, have a fence or something that blocks somebody from coming up to the house at all. Unfortunately, there are many mentally, emotionally, and sexually unwell people today. Do not let your children become a victim. Especially today, you need to take extra precautions with your kids' access to technology. A cell phone is the only window a predator needs to begin luring and peeping on them in this day and age. Be vigilant. And check yourself constantly with what you allow across your own screens.

You Get to Move On from That

Whatever trauma you have experienced, you get to move on. It doesn't get to hold you hostage. There is tremendous freedom from getting through it.

With any trauma, how can you reframe what happened? How can you heal? And in what ways can you find forgiveness? Even from a human perspective, how can you approach rather than avoid . . . using the trauma in a new way.

Otherwise, it feels like holding a pipe that is starting to burst open. And once one starts, then all the other pipes start bursting around you. Because we know that what you resist persists. If you feel like you are avoiding it, remember that you might be missing out on the miracle of life if you are only looking at the horror show.

Resistance

When I first started sharing my story, I felt a lot of internal resistance. I was invited to speak about my experiences on the *Shawn Ryan Show*, and it one of the most challenging things I have ever done in my whole life. I am grateful to him for providing the safe space for me to share my story with others who may be in a similar position so they can know they are not alone.

My purpose is to show what is possible by sharing my journey and at the same time, I hate being the center of attention. When I was first invited to do the show, I knew that I had to do it. If my story can help just one person, it's worth it to break through the resistance.

If there is anything that comes to mind to anyone who reads this, know that you are not alone. Most of the things I hear about from people happened before they were 18. I hear more and more often from people I am connecting with that something happened to them, or to somebody they know or care about. If this is you, know that you are not alone and there are ways to work through this trauma. There are resources for support.

The more that I find ways to break the silence, share my story, and see the impact it has on others, the more I know that I am living in my purpose. I just have to remember to keep my focus faced outward.

Before going on the show, I was anxious, knowing that I was going to be asked about certain areas of my life that I hadn't talked publicly about before. It created a lot of stress and anxiety for at least a month before the interview. I kept telling myself that if it helps one person get through a tough time, it's worth doing.

The episode aired five months later, and the response was more than I ever expected. Thousands of people from all walks of life have reached out since it aired to let me know what resonated with them or helped them break through something that was bothering them.

Looking back, I'm extremely grateful for the healing that the experience created for others and for myself. I feel a hundred pounds lighter from letting go of some of the old memories that came up.

If you have a powerful story or experience that may help others. Do *not* hold back. Tell your story and share your experience in the medium that's right for you, because you never know who is going to hear it and be affected by it.

Stop Feeding the Bad Wolf

A Native American parable teaches that two wolves live within us: one represents negativity, fear, and ego, while the other embodies kindness, courage, and love. The wolf that thrives is the one you feed. Choose carefully which thoughts and actions you nourish.

> One evening, an elderly Cherokee brave told his grandson about a battle that goes on inside people.
>
> He said, "My son, the battle is between two 'wolves' inside us all. One is evil. It is anger, envy, jealousy, sorrow, regret, greed, arrogance, self-pity, guilt, resentment, inferiority, lies, false pride, superiority, and ego.
>
> The other is good. It is joy, peace, love, hope, serenity, humility, kindness, benevolence, empathy, generosity, truth, compassion, and faith."
>
> The grandson thought about it for a minute and then asked his grandfather, "Which wolf wins?"
>
> The old Cherokee simply replied, "The one that you feed."

Create Deep Meaning in Life

I've been in these different modes of scarcity throughout my life. But now, I am in a place of flow and abundance with my relationships, family, kids, dogs, work team, mentors, and the different activities I get to do.

My favorite thing in life that also brings me meaning and extreme joy is seeing people around me succeed and break through glass ceilings to unlock their dreams.

I had to do that for myself first. I grew up along the ocean and always longed to surf. I had driven by jiu jitsu gyms, watched fighting and different martial arts since I was a kid. I always wanted to see if I could do those things. Now, I've been surfing and training in martial arts for a few years. They help me unlock full creativity and flow. Now that I am doing these things, I think about what else is possible. These activities unlock a lot of creativity and possibilities because I am mastering and developing all these skills that I always desired.

Whatever it is that is calling you to try or experience in your life, I encourage you to approach it and see how these actions can make small and big changes in your life.

Create a Positive Shift

When I was finishing my undergraduate degree, my final paper was about Latin American culture. I had studied about all these different types of cultures. My big takeaway from this assignment is that once cultures are set, it is not easy or even possible to make immediate changes to them. But what you can do is create shifts. Then you can create waves. These waves lead to lasting change.

With everything going on in the world with technology, the second and third order effects of everything that happened or failed to happen since COVID, and how human resiliency is today, we want to be what is missing within the culture. We want to be the positive shift. Even with DEF and Underwater Torpedo League, people resisted at first, saying things like, "Oh, this is too dangerous . . . ." We haven't had any injuries or claims, and we are helping people shatter their glass ceilings and find new levels of what is possible and human performance. Now, the feedback is more like, "Wow, these people are holding their breath for minutes . . . is that possible for me?" We love to see those breakthroughs open the door for more people to build resiliency.

For anyone who participates in the programs, what we find is that anxiety and depression significantly decrease, and mental health improve. That's just from the mental health side. Athletes training underwater with us at DEF are achieving unprecedented fitness levels, which creates a uniquely supportive community. Our driving force is to expand this positive impact nationwide and globally.

Relationship with Higher Power

When I was having all my mental health breakdowns in 2018–2019, I was focused a lot on myself. There wasn't a focus on God or my spirituality. I've always believed in Him and leaned on Him. But there were times when I've fallen off. I want to emphasize that when I talk about plant medicine or any other approaches toward healing, **none of it works without God in my life**.

The word *God* is incredibly complex, and as humans, it can be hard to fully understand what it means. That's why personal experience matters so much. We come to know God through what we live, not by following someone else's version of faith. I didn't find God in church. I first found Him in a closet, when I was alone, isolated, and searching for safety. In those quiet moments, something would come over me. A sense of calm I never felt sitting in a pew. That was the beginning of my real connection with a higher power, and it has stayed personal ever since.

It's Pandora's box when you begin to unpack traumas and ask questions. But once my spiritual awareness and I had a moment of active surrender to God, and I became in tune with God's plan is for me, I know I want to live that plan the best that I can.

What I noticed is that when I had those first spiritual experiences, it was the strongest and closest to God I have ever felt, and it brought me to a new level of letting go. I didn't have that spiritual awareness yet. I wasn't taking the time to review the information coming in, look for the lesson, and ask God what He wants me to do.

Looking back at all the ways my life could have ended, even back to the first time I fractured my skull, to being jumped, in car accidents or being hit in insider attacks, if something had gone just slightly different, I could have died in any of those situations. So, every day, I'm grateful to be alive and walking around. I know I am blessed to have my family, friends, purpose, job, and the role in the world that I do. God kept me and graced me with the ability to make it through each challenge so I can make an impact with others and be a light in the world. And I am committed to doing that as much as I can.

I believe that all things are possible with God. My relationship with God is the most important thing to me. Nothing I do matters without Him. And at the end of the day, the plant medicine opened my ability to have a relationship with God; it was not a replacement for that relationship.

Spirituality was always something in the back of my mind. I was so focused on all the wrong things that it got crowded out. I didn't have any practices aside from small prayers. Plant medicine helped open that pathway for me in many ways, and after that, I started reading and studying the Bible. I am a white belt with the Bible. I feel like a little kid reading it, but the messages that I get from it are strong. The version of the Bible that I am reading was one I took with me on my deployments. It was issued to us from the chaplain, the cover is camouflage and fits into your pocket. I have since become interested in the contents of the Bible and curious about it. Why are there so many different versions? What may or may not be missing from the versions we have today?

A lot of people have religious or spiritual trauma that creates resistance. I had bad experiences with church growing up. My priest, who was the priest of the whole church that I went to as a kid, was also a part-time mime and clown. We would go on these retreats, and he would go into the other room and change into these outfits and then would come out and scare us. There was something off/horrifying with this man. It reminds me now of that horror movie *IT*. You could tell he was disturbed. He would turn into the mime and do strange hand and body motions . . . and he was the priest of the church.

I got confirmed when I was 12 and I had to go to these summer camps. The priest was banned from them while I was going. His two children had both committed suicide. Every Sunday I had to sit in church with him until after my parents divorced. These experiences were traumatizing and gave me a resistance to church environments. It was hard for me to get into church after that. I had no interest.

Just like with anything, if you are not open to receive information, you will not be open to it and will not mean anything to you when it comes your way. But when I became open to it, I realized it's fascinating.

There are so many strange traditions we celebrate without really thinking. Near Halloween, I go on early morning jogs and am startled by lawn decorations that scream or jump out when I pass by. It triggers my post-traumatic stress response, even if only for a moment. I often wonder why we normalize things that are designed to scare us.

I try to think critically about the world around me and question what we are taught to accept. A more countercultural path has always felt more honest. If I didn't run a business or need to stay connected to other people, I probably wouldn't carry a phone. It often feels more like a leash than a tool.

How imperfect we all are as humans. Everybody gets grace and forgiveness from God and if God can forgive us, we can forgive other people and ultimately forgive ourselves.

CHAPTER 13

Wavetops

During my final eight years of military service, debriefings were sometimes a daily occurrence. This practice extended even to training scenarios, when life-threatening situations could arise. To ensure that critical failures were documented and lessons were promptly learned, we were instructed to "just focus on the wave tops," which meant to drive home the key takeaways and not to go down rabbit holes or get lost in small details that don't create immediate solutions.

Writing *Permission to Heal* has allowed me to reflect on a lot. I wanted to share the biggest takeaways or wave tops from my experiences to bring everything full circle. This chapter is built differently from the other chapters in that it flows from concept to concept. This is meant to provide a high-level overview and reference guide for me to share some of my most important realizations and takeaways that I have seen unlock the most performance in my own life and those in my circle.

Reframing

It's important to note that not every day is going to be easy breezy and that there will not be breakdowns along the way. When times get tough, focus out and remember that even a broken clock is right twice a day. Can you look at your current challenge in a different way? What are two things that you could get right today that could shift something in your life or in the life of someone else in a positive direction?

Ego/Relationship with Self

Letting go of the old me that wanted to ego flex, allowing myself to show up differently, was the most important thing I ever did. Try to look at good ego versus bad ego. Good ego comes from love and spiritual guidance. Emotional intelligence (EQ) training and coaching can support you in regulating your emotions and building a higher understanding of what emotions drive your actions. Equally important is understanding what emotions drive others you engage with, so you can come from a better place of understanding and not from a place of judgment.

Letting Go of Attachments

Chuck Palahniuk, author of *Fight Club*, has said, "The things you own end up owning you. It's only when we have lost everything that we are free to do anything."

Somebody who gets out of the military and has a lot of rank is a textbook example of someone with attachments. Because when they get out, they have no rank. Your previous rank doesn't matter when you are out. Nobody cares what you achieved or accomplished. Letting go of the attachment to the rank can be incredibly difficult.

Most of my young adult life was spent living out of a backpack. I was always gone, my belongings were always in storage, and I was constantly traveling. My stuff was never organized in a home. I had items in multiple storage units. Finally, when Brittany and I got our house, I got everything all set up and organized. It was a special feeling when I was finally able to do this.

We ended up selling this house during the pandemic, living in a trailer, and camping on the beach and at cool camp sites until things started to "normalize" again after a year and a half. We were happier in this tiny trailer than we ever were in the big house. Once we were able to let go of the comfort of living in the house and the attachments to our belongings, it ended up being the best. My daughter Hanna talks about when we lived in the camper all the time. I learned through this that sometimes you need to give to get. You need to give up attachment to your material things to get different types of peace and freedom that comes with letting go and detaching from all the things.

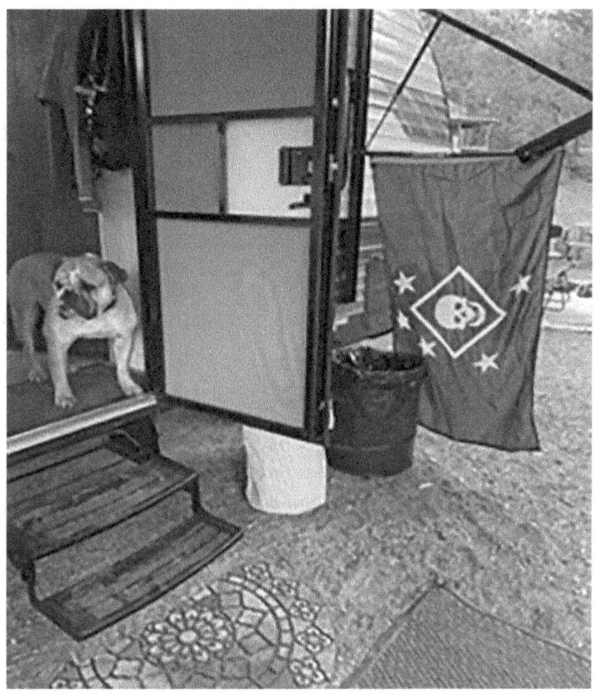

Camper life during Covid 2020–2021

At my last house, we had TVs in every room in the house. When we moved into a normal house again, we only put one TV up. Shortly after, we took it out. It's been a game changer and it's so nice to see the kids playing games, cards, and reading books. The connection that a lack of technology brings is priceless to me. Crazy to think that in most modern households, *people spend significant amounts of time in their own room in the house, on their smartphone, and feel isolated.*

Surrendering Versus Quitting

Surrendering is all about *letting go.* It's about letting your old self surrender or dissolve and letting go of the past. The challenge is attachments to memories and stories you have about yourself. A lot of it is egocentric. Let go of attachments and surrender the ego. It's okay to have ego, but learning to have a healthy relationship with it is key. Give allowance for new beginnings and radical acceptance.

I used to have this never-quit mentality built in, which did not work at a certain point. Understand the difference between quitting and surrendering. Being able to quit when things are not working for you anymore is important, and surrendering to be open to new possibilities requires letting go of resistance. Being in a beginner's mindset is what allows new possibilities.

Limiting Beliefs

Limiting beliefs are like programs in our operating system that hold us back from our highest potential and self. They are some of the biggest factors I have experienced myself and have seen with my family, friends, coaching clients—anyone—from making progress on any front.

When I was younger, I was told I was a bad kid, and I was in trouble a lot. My first Marine Corps recruiter told me there was no way I could get into the military with my criminal record. When I got out of the marines I was medically separated and was told by my military doctors that I wasn't going to be able to run or do a lot of activities that I enjoyed and that I would not be able to function without a bag of medications. These are just two examples of limiting beliefs or barriers I've experienced that I now realize were holding me back in life. The people we surround ourselves with, the things we tell ourselves, all our memories, can sometimes build these limiting beliefs and create stories that hold us back. What action can you take to identify and eliminate one limiting belief to break through to the next level?

Circle of Trust: Tribe, Community, Coaches

With trusted people in your corner and a strong why, you can do hard things. Remove cancerous people from your circle as soon as you can—pull those weeds. It is important to take time and energy to build and water our relationships—with our higher power, self, family, friends, and others, as well as our relationship with nature.

Finding Your Why

If you struggle with defining your why, look to the people closest to you in your life.

Consider those closest to you when defining your why. Imagine a tree of life with three branches: family, friends, and teachers/coaches.

- Now that you've framed out the most important relationships in your circle. What makes you a contributing member to this tribe?
- What is your superpower and how does this serve others?
- What does everyone know about you that you don't know about yourself?
- What are you pretending not to know about yourself, your value, and how you can contribute?

Crows and Eagles

You rise and fall to the quality of the people around you. I think of the story of the eagle when a crow comes and disturbs it. Instead of attacking the crow, the eagle starts to soar to higher altitudes. If you are high performing and there are people coming around who hold you back, soar to a higher level and they will just fall off. Sometimes in life, people talk nonstop, pestering you with things you're not interest in. But actions always speak louder than words. Just soar, move to a higher altitude and see who stays with you. Your true friends will show themselves when times get tough. Good buddies are like flashlights or night vision when you are in darkness.

Alcohol (or Other)

Let go of whatever it is that creates a barrier and holds you back.

My key to healing and personal growth has been consistently abstaining from alcohol. While my struggle was with alcohol, for others this could manifest as an overreliance on medications. I've observed this pattern repeatedly in my own life and among family and friends. Initially, my goal was 10 years without drinking, but now it extends from my first 5-MeO-DMT experience. Consider what you might eliminate from your own life.

If you think about it, what is the thing that you can remove from your life?

Close Out Unnecessary Tabs

You only have so much bandwidth, cognitive horsepower, or whatever you want to call it. Focus on the things that really matter to you and your well-being and close out the tabs that create drag for you and limit your performance.

Unlock more mental flow with a clear mind, one that is free of clutter and focused on one tab. Less is more. If you constantly try to chase multiple rabbits, you will catch none of them.

What is it that you can remove from your life that would change it significantly for the better? If you did this, what would your life look like in six months, one year, five years from now?

What can you eliminate from your life that would get you closer to your goals or create a breakthrough for you? For example, Would removing TVs from your house or apps from your phone benefit you? Do you need better boundaries with your phone? Do you have habits or patterns like drinking or going to clubs? Or eating unhealthy foods?

Isolate yourself from the things that are holding you back.

"When I Am Better, They Are Better"

It's been almost five years since I went on that first healing journey. It was scary to do it but I didn't have any other options at that point. The spiritual lessons and integrations that *one* experience brought were lifelong and life changing. Before this experience, I was not on speaking terms with a lot of my family members. I had problems with almost everybody. The healing and subsequent integration work has allowed me to restore a lot of those relationships. Recently, I coordinated a reunion on my dad's side of the family. On my mom's side, we've connected a lot more spiritually and many of those family members have approached plant medicines as well.

You never know the ripple effect that you taking care of yourself or healing yourself will have on everyone around you. Or any health or self-improvement you do. Or when you max out your potential. *Uni verse* means "one song," and it is important to remember that we are all connected and we all come from the same creator.

Love over Fear

We all have egos and experience times when people attack us, and we want to respond or react in a way that is not aligned with our highest self. This can put us into a low vibrational state.

I have seen a lot of situations where the only thing that could solve a dispute was love. There can't be fear that lives in the same space as love. It can be hard to find that place of love. But I am a prime example of what's possible, because at one point I was in a state of conflict with almost everybody. These days, it's the opposite. For the most part, my relationships are working, but I still have a few I struggle with that I continue to work on.

Some relationships are meant to end. And there will be new beginnings with new relationships that form. Sometimes there's more grace that is needed for that individual, especially if they are in a bad place. When someone operates from a place of desperation, they might be a narcissist, gas lighting others and other such behaviors. The worst thing to do is to give it attention or focus. You don't need to give it any energy. Let that go and let love into the equation. Find and accept the highest vibration of love.

I've learned and am learning this that if you hold onto resentment, you are poisoning yourself and expecting the other person to die. You are just hurting yourself. Do whatever you can to open your ability to love.

The breakdown and tragedy of it all is to see all the people who are committing suicide and the wars that break out. I try to see the silver lining in such tragedies. People are waking up more. People are more open to making positive change.

The veteran community is a good example. Five to 10 years ago, it was all about ego. Ego is a necessary part of the job and culture in special operations to an extent and always has been that way. We still embraced the "suffer in silence" culture. Thankfully the culture is shifting away from this mentality, but it has taken a lot of our people dying for us to reach this level of empathy as a community.

Now when people get together, they look out for each other. Check on each other. Be a good person and human to each other. Recently I am seeing and hearing from a lot more of my old teammates and people I served with. This is a good sign, and I am hopeful that the veteran community will continue to work together to create solutions for each other. How can we get together more, stay connected, do something positive for the community? How can we get fewer guys to kill themselves this year than last year?

Water Is Life

How we react to the water is how we react to life. How we do one thing we do all things. As I've described, the two biomechanics of swimming are increasing propulsion and reducing friction—increasing flow while reducing drag. The lessons I've learned and shared in this book also are the foundation for the cultural ethos of Deep End Fitness (DEF) and Underwater Torpedo League (UTL).

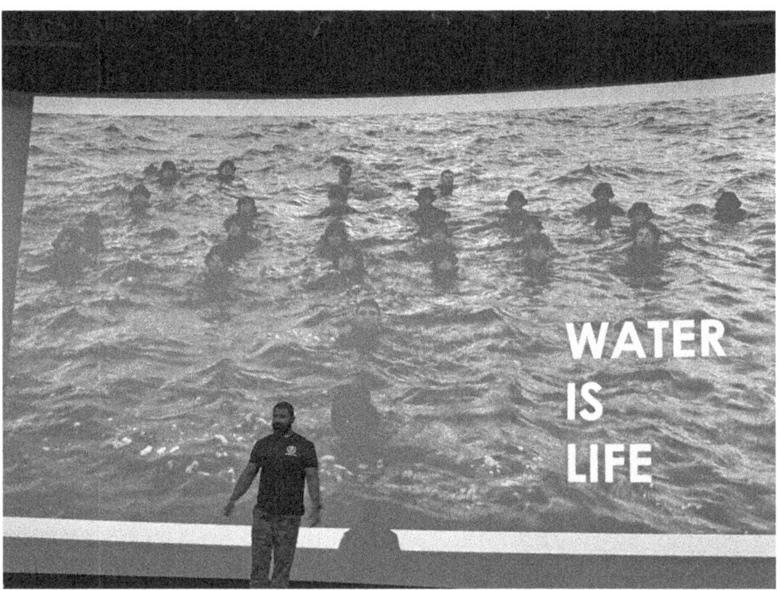

Prime Speaking to the Marines at Camp Pendleton, California (2024)

An organization's cultural ethos is one of its most important aspects. When I speak, I talk about our cultural ethos in the following ways:

◆ DEF is a merit-based organization. Athletes are 100% responsible for their own performance and growth.

◆ Obstacles promote growth. Progress cannot be made in the comfort zone.

- DEF has a "no flex zone" environment. The standards are set in the circle of trust.
- The buddy/guardian system is always in effect.
- We respect each other, the water, and the sport at all times.
- Our training mantra is "calm breeds calm."
- Everything we do is to benefit the team, which in turn empowers each individual.
- We do not compromise safety standards for the sake of growth.
- We operate off of brilliance in the basics, from the acronym F.R.E.E. (focus, relaxation, economy of motion, efficient breathing).
- What is said in the circle of trust remains in the circle of trust.

Be Brave Enough to Face the War in Your Mind

Since I started sharing my story, a marine general at Camp Pendleton brought me back on base and positioned me to be on a speaking circuit that could include some swimming pool (DEF) activations along with a leadership/resilience talk that provides tools and frameworks for performance, mindset, breath-work tools, and more all within a two-hour block. We've since launched a new resilience program in the Marine Corps. When I was first asked to speak, the organizers said I was like a modern-day Jack Matthews, and my story was relatable to so many.

Being compared to Jack Matthews, the person who inspired me during my struggles, feels like a full-circle moment. It's been an incredible opportunity to pay forward the impact he had on me. This wouldn't have been possible without introspection and confronting my own thoughts with the support of my family, friends, and coaches.

Illusions

Dominick Cruz shared this:

"One of the biggest illusions we all have, is that (1) we are all separate, and (2) we are not suffering." Everyone tries to put on a front, but every person I know is suffering or dealing with something. Our ego puts on this illusion that we are the only one dealing with anything. What we're dealing with is different. Every person is dealing with their own issues, and they are attached or holding onto something that they have not dealt with or processed. But none of us know that, especially when we get isolated and get in our own head. And that's when that illusion gets stronger and stronger that we are in this all by ourselves, but when in reality, everyone suffers along in their journey.

I have seen good friends feel as if they have lost their minds and have issues with their mental health. Everyone is dealing with something. And it's only because I engage with so many veterans that I see these patterns. But when I look at other groups, I see it just as clearly. It's almost black and white with veterans. A lot of us are dealing with the same thing; we just don't know it because we are not communicating to others about our vulnerabilities, *but we all have them.*

Others have their own traumas from life. I can relate to all these different people, and we all can overcome our traumas if we put intention behind it.

Open or Closed Mindset

Zen master Shunryu Suzuki is supposed to have said, "In the beginner's mind there are many possibilities, but in the expert's mind there are few."

Are you open in general?

Are you open to receiving abundance in your life?

Are you open to receiving love?

Are you open to receiving honest feedback?

I learned a lot about this at an EQ course in Las Vegas. We had to do these long hugs, like in *Fight Club*. There is this scene in the movie where Edward Norton's character is crying on the shoulder of the character Bob in a self-help group. This reminds me of some of my experiences in the EQ course. When we first did this, I wanted to jump out of my skin. What I learned about myself was that I was really closed off and in resistance. With those experiences, plus my healing work, I am now open to feedback.

It's easy to stay in a fixed mindset. It might be in our nature as humans to gravitate toward a fixed mindset, because that means we stay safe. Sometimes you have to challenge yourself to stay open. That's the path to continue learning and evolving. Are you open or closed off? Are you in an open mindset? Are you in a beginner's mindset? From my experience, it takes intention and commitment to evolve and grow as a person to remain open in life.

Since I first tried the plant medicine, I have noticed a lot more of my blind spots. Similarly, when I went to those EQ courses, which I did for a couple of years, they really showed my blind spots. I've seen sides of myself I didn't see before. What I learned about myself was that I was in resistance and in a closed mindset. I thought because I went through all these crazy trainings and experiences in the military, and even before that, that I knew a lot. I didn't.

Another big realization I had while attending these courses is that throughout my military training, I had been in a couple of interrogation trainings that taught me a lot about resistance. Little did I know that those resistance techniques were holding me back in civilian life. I was in resistance with almost everything in modern society if I allowed myself to be. Or I could *shift* and allow myself to surrender this resistance and be intentional with my thoughts and energy.

Giving and Receiving

Everything is an energy exchange. I realized that I had a blockage about receiving. I see this with other people who will over give and do a lot for other people, but don't take care of themselves enough. They can give, but they also must learn to receive; otherwise, there is a blockage in the natural loop of giving and receiving.

Be What's Missing

When you look at a relationship, especially when there is a conflict or misunderstanding, ask yourself *What is missing?* in that situation. Is it love? If so, then try to be loving or be what's missing. Is communication missing? What gap needs to be filled to unlock flow? However, if what you have to offer isn't moving a problem or situation forward, if you can't be what's missing, be missing. Walk away.

Talk Versus Show

Actions speak louder than words. Always. Especially when you are in a bind or in a challenging situation.

When we started UTL, we tried to explain to people what the sport was and what our vision was, but they'd look at us confused. Then we'd pull up a video and show them. Suddenly, their eyes would light up. You could see the switch flip. They didn't need more explanation. We didn't have to break it down any further. The visual did it all. That one moment communicated more than an hour of explanation ever could. Showing and modeling something to somebody garners exponentially more results than just talking about something.

Discernment: Smoke and Mirrors

Discernment is the ability to see through smoke and mirrors, and the ability to detect what's authentic, genuine, and rooted in good intentions versus what's false or misleading. It's about recognizing red flags when something feels off or appears dishonest. Trust your instincts when things don't align and always use your discernment. We're entering an age where reality itself can be uncertain. This underscores how critical it is to approach everything in life with discernment. In a world where it's increasingly hard to tell what's real, intentionality becomes essential. Don't drift through life aimlessly or surround yourself with people who don't align with your values. Take accountability. Design your life with purpose. Take control and use discernment to ensure everything in your life serves you and your vision.

From the Darkness into the Light

Sometimes light come out of the darkness. As my wife says, "From the darkness, into the light." I have experienced heavy darkness in my life and now I am operating in the light. I am mission oriented to not only spread light in the world but also to wake people up who might be asleep.

My vision for the world is world peace by 2030. I envision a world that mutually supports each other and promotes truth and collaboration with all of humanity.

Success isn't about avoiding challenges but about navigating them intentionally. Design a life that prioritizes growth, authenticity, and meaningful relationships while clearing the noise that distracts from your purpose.

I never wanted to write a book about myself mainly because I never wanted to put myself out there and expose my vulnerability. That all changed when a handful of my friends and brothers whom I served with took their lives, and seeing so many people I know and care about struggle with mental health. What I have learned is that almost every person I know seems to be struggling with something, in some kind of battle in their own lives. I feel like we are all connected with each other, and not so different from one another. I hope that this book affects everyone who reads it in a positive way, not just to support unlocking flow and removing drag from their lives but to provide tools for self-regulation, coping, and shifting and reframing pain into purpose.

This book comes from a very humble place, in the trenches, as Don said in the Foreword. My intent and hope are that this book helps you break through something meaningful for you in your life.

Remember when you feel like you can't move and are stuck, try to crawl. Start crawling until you are able to walk. Walk until you can run. Run until you can fly.

Through the darkness there is light. Stay in the flow.

With love,

Prime

P.S. Never let the world take your smile.

Resources

For the full list of resources and books, visit www.PrimeHall.com.

Acknowledgments

To my wife Brittany and amazing kids Trey and Hanna—thank you for inspiring me to grow spiritually, mentally, and emotionally.

To all my family members: Hall, Burns, Rusteberg, and Fordyce, and all our ancestors.

To my parents, for giving me life and the opportunity to grow. Without you, none of this story would be possible.

To Nana, Papa, Aunt Christy and Uncle Steve, Aunt Kathy, Uncle Will, Aunt Frances and all my amazing cousins Jake, Ben, Jessie Rose, Bill, Austin, Sarita and my Goddaughter Marilyn Belle—I love you all very much.

To Brittany's family, Leezy, Gary, Alex, Di, Ashley, Chris, Zach and Meg.

Don, I wouldn't have made it through Raider training I don't think without you, and Deep End Fitness (DEF) and Underwater Torpedo League (UTL) wouldn't be possible without you. Thanks for always being what's missing and a rock.

Derek for being an amazing mentor and positive example. Ricky and Derek for being the miracles with what happened on June 14, 2012, in Afghanistan. From almost losing both of you, to everything that we have done since we got out of the military.

To all the amazing mentors and support circle. To all members of the DEF and UTL community that has been a huge why to keep us going when we need it.

Dom for always holding me accountable with how I am showing up in the world for myself and for others. I am grateful for all the deep and meaningful conversations we get to have.

Ricky Briere for being a ride or die friend and sticking with me over the years to me and my family.

Myles for being relentless with me until I got into healing and all the work that you continue to do.

To Rodie for dedicating so much time and energy to the positive growth and healing of others and their families. We are all grateful to have you in our corner.

Ryan Spadafore for fostering the closeness with our community and tribe, and keeping the dream alive.

My integration therapist, Dr. Michelle, who told me the first time I met her that I would write several books.

Bethany for taking this project on and deep diving some of the hardest subjects and experiences that I've had and being an amazing support through all of it. Thank you for your dedication to this mission. Thank you to Leah, Julie, and the Wiley publishing team.

To all our investors, supporters, and amazing community members of DEF and UTL. Without you all, the dream would not have been possible.

All my teammates and brave souls whom I had the privilege of serving with—this book is especially for you.

To all of those who made the ultimate sacrifice.

About the Author

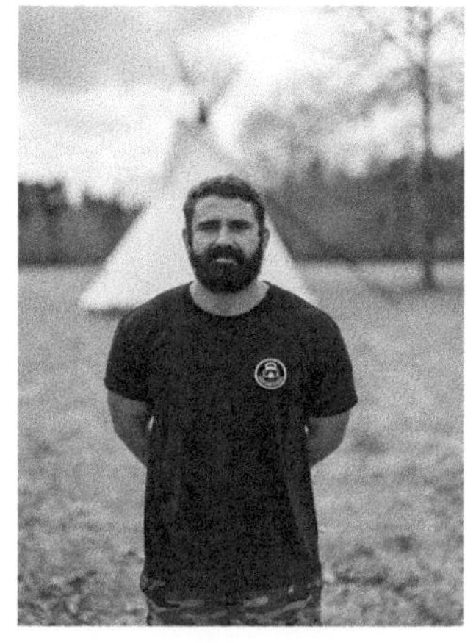

Prime Hall grew up in Texas, where he attended the Marine Military Academy. A few years later he entered the marine infantry before advancing as a MARSOC Marine Raider, with a specialty as a Marine Corps Instructor of Water Survival. He uses tools and techniques, which he brings from this background, as well as what he has learned from training thousands of individuals and teams to create personal breakthroughs. His *F.R.E.E. Your Mind Guidebook* is the result of these findings, in which a framework was created to coach world-class athletes, business executives, and military special operations candidates looking to perform at a higher level. The immediate result has been a powerful shift in their lives. Prime's goal is to facilitate lasting life changes with as many people as possible who, in turn, will create a better society. Prime is a human potential coach and cofounder of the Underwater Torpedo League and Deep End Fitness. Prime currently resides in Southern California.

Index